CONTENTS

Page

Testimony of:

Azar, Hon. Alex M., Deputy Secretary, U.S. Department of Health and Human Services 8

O'Toole, Dr. Tara, CEO and Director, Center for Biosecurity, The University of Pittsburgh Medical Center 33

Young, Peter F., President and CEO, AlphaVax, Inc., on behalf of Biotechnology Industry Organization 41

Cohen, Bruce, President and CEO, Cellerant Therapeutics, Inc. 48

Wright, Dr. David P., President and CEO, PharmAthene, on behalf of Alliance for Biosecurity 53

Blaser, Dr. Martin, President, Infectious Diseases Society of America 59

Additional material submitted for the record:

Azar, Hon. Alex M., Deputy Secretary, U.S. Department of Health and Human Services, response for the record 78

PROJECT BIOSHIELD REAUTHORIZATION ISSUES

HEARING

BEFORE THE

SUBCOMMITTEE ON HEALTH

OF THE

COMMITTEE ON ENERGY AND COMMERCE
HOUSE OF REPRESENTATIVES

ONE HUNDRED NINTH CONGRESS

SECOND SESSION

APRIL 6, 2006

Serial No. 109-97

Printed for the use of the Committee on Energy and Commerce

Available via the World Wide Web: http://www.access.gpo.gov/congress/house

---

U.S. GOVERNMENT PRINTING OFFICE

29-726PDF WASHINGTON : 2006

For sale by the Superintendent of Documents, U.S. Government Printing Office
Internet: bookstore.gpo.gov Phone: toll free (866) 512-1800; DC area (202) 512-1800
Fax: (202) 512-2250 Mail: Stop SSOP, Washington, DC 20402-0001

COMMITTEE ON ENERGY AND COMMERCE

JOE BARTON, Texas, *Chairman*

RALPH M. HALL, Texas
MICHAEL BILIRAKIS, Florida
Vice Chairman
FRED UPTON, Michigan
CLIFF STEARNS, Florida
PAUL E. GILLMOR, Ohio
NATHAN DEAL, Georgia
ED WHITFIELD, Kentucky
CHARLIE NORWOOD, Georgia
BARBARA CUBIN, Wyoming
JOHN SHIMKUS, Illinois
HEATHER WILSON, New Mexico
JOHN B. SHADEGG, Arizona
CHARLES W. "CHIP" PICKERING, Mississippi
Vice Chairman
VITO FOSSELLA, New York
ROY BLUNT, Missouri
STEVE BUYER, Indiana
GEORGE RADANOVICH, California
CHARLES F. BASS, New Hampshire
JOSEPH R. PITTS, Pennsylvania
MARY BONO, California
GREG WALDEN, Oregon
LEE TERRY, Nebraska
MIKE FERGUSON, New Jersey
MIKE ROGERS, Michigan
C.L. "BUTCH" OTTER, Idaho
SUE MYRICK, North Carolina
JOHN SULLIVAN, Oklahoma
TIM MURPHY, Pennsylvania
MICHAEL C. BURGESS, Texas
MARSHA BLACKBURN, Tennessee

JOHN D. DINGELL, Michigan
Ranking Member
HENRY A. WAXMAN, California
EDWARD J. MARKEY, Massachusetts
RICK BOUCHER, Virginia
EDOLPHUS TOWNS, New York
FRANK PALLONE, JR., New Jersey
SHERROD BROWN, Ohio
BART GORDON, Tennessee
BOBBY L. RUSH, Illinois
ANNA G. ESHOO, California
BART STUPAK, Michigan
ELIOT L. ENGEL, New York
ALBERT R. WYNN, Maryland
GENE GREEN, Texas
TED STRICKLAND, Ohio
DIANA DEGETTE, Colorado
LOIS CAPPS, California
MIKE DOYLE, Pennsylvania
TOM ALLEN, Maine
JIM DAVIS, Florida
JAN SCHAKOWSKY, Illinois
HILDA L. SOLIS, California
CHARLES A. GONZALEZ, Texas
JAY INSLEE, Washington
TAMMY BALDWIN, Wisconsin
MIKE ROSS, Arkansas

BUD ALBRIGHT, *Staff Director*
DAVID CAVICKE, *General Counsel*
REID P. F. STUNTZ, *Minority Staff Director and Chief Counsel*

SUBCOMMITTEE ON HEALTH

NATHAN DEAL, Georgia, *Chairman*

RALPH M. HALL, Texas
MICHAEL BILIRAKIS, Florida
FRED UPTON, Michigan
PAUL E. GILLMOR, Ohio
CHARLIE NORWOOD, Georgia
BARBARA CUBIN, Wyoming
JOHN SHIMKUS, Illinois
JOHN B. SHADEGG, Arizona
CHARLES W. "CHIP" PICKERING, Mississippi
STEVE BUYER, Indiana
JOSEPH R. PITTS, Pennsylvania
MARY BONO, California
MIKE FERGUSON, New Jersey
MIKE ROGERS, Michigan
SUE MYRICK, North Carolina
MICHAEL C. BURGESS, Texas
JOE BARTON, Texas
(EX OFFICIO)

SHERROD BROWN, Ohio
Ranking Member
HENRY A. WAXMAN, California
EDOLPHUS TOWNS, New York
FRANK PALLONE, JR., New Jersey
BART GORDON, Tennessee
BOBBY L. RUSH, Illinois
ANNA G. ESHOO, California
GENE GREEN, Texas
TED STRICKLAND, Ohio
DIANA DEGETTE, Colorado
LOIS CAPPS, California
TOM ALLEN, Maine
JIM DAVIS, Florida
TAMMY BALDWIN, Wisconsin
JOHN D. DINGELL, Michigan
(EX OFFICIO)

PROJECT BIOSHIELD REAUTHORIZATION ISSUES

THURSDAY, APRIL 6, 2006

HOUSE OF REPRESENTATIVES,
COMMITTEE ON ENERGY AND COMMERCE,
SUBCOMMITTEE ON HEALTH,
Washington, DC.

The subcommittee met, pursuant to notice, at 1:02 p.m., in Room 2123 of the Rayburn House Office Building, Hon. Nathan Deal (chairman) presiding.

Members present: Representatives Deal, Cubin, Shimkus, Rogers, Myrick, Burgess, Pallone, Eshoo, and Green.

Staff present: David Rosenfeld, Acting Chief Health Counsel; Ryan Long, Counsel; Nandan Kenkeremath, Counsel; Bill O'Brien, Legislative Analyst; Brandon Clark, Policy Coordinator; Chad Grant, Legislative Clerk; John Ford, Minority Counsel; and Jessica McNiece, Minority Research Assistant.

MR. DEAL. We are pleased to have a very special group of individuals to testify before the committee today on two separate panels. Today, we are going to be reviewing one of the critical pieces of our biodefense structure. This committee has important responsibilities in this area and has passed a number of pieces of legislation to deal with chemical, biological, radiological, and nuclear threats. I want to commend the leadership of the President in leading the way on pandemic flu preparedness and biodefense preparedness. I know activities are underway at multiple Departments, including HHS, the Department of Homeland Security, and the Department of Defense, dealing with these issues. A great deal has been done with respect to the first round of material threats as defined by the Department of Homeland Security. There are many continuing questions about how to access threats, whether these should include naturally occurring threats, and how to develop an appropriate response.

We want to make sure that the various Departments and offices are properly coordinating and have the right expertise. We know that biodefense is an area where the Federal government must take a strong role. There is no business model that will support the investments we need without a clear path from the Federal government. We also know that the expertise is in the private sector, so we must make sure that we have a working partnership there as well. We want to work closely with

HHS and other agencies to improve Project BioShield and our overall pandemic and bioterrorism preparedness. I thank our witnesses for their attendance today and we will look forward to hearing their testimony, beginning with the first panel as soon as we complete the opening statements.

MR. DEAL. I will now recognize my friend, Mr. Pallone from New Jersey, for his opening statement.

MR. PALLONE. Thank you, Mr. Chairman, and thanks also to the witnesses for participating in today's hearing and I know the subcommittee is eager to hear your testimony. Nearly two years ago Congress passed the Project BioShield Act with tremendous bipartisan support. Democrats and Republicans worked together to establish a process that would help our Nation respond to bioterrorism threats and attacks. Today's hearing will give us an opportunity to assess how well the program is working to meet this important goal.

Since going into effect, a number of criticisms have been make against the program and much of that criticism has come from the biotech industry and has been leveled against the Department of Homeland Security and the Department of Health and Human Services. The complaint I hear most often is that the Federal government has been too slow to assess bioterrorism threats and award contracts to the acquisition of effective countermeasures. Now the Homeland Security Department has been accused of taking too long to issue material threat determinations, which is needed before Health and Human Services can acquire necessary countermeasures. And while this may be a legitimate criticism, as I understand it, even if DHS were to provide these assessments in a more timely manner, HHS currently lacks the necessary resources to take appropriate action. Indeed, it is not clear to me that the current organizational structure or staffing levels at HHS are adequate to provide for the timely acquisition of effective countermeasures, and I would certainly be interested to hear from Mr. Azar. I think I heard them name Mr. Azar on this subject.

Furthermore, I am not certain that those at HHS charged with administering the program have the proper background or expertise to successfully carry out its mission. For example, Mr. Chairman, I don't think it is in the best interests of the country to have an Assistant Secretary of Public Health Emergency Preparedness who has no background in public health or emergency preparedness, and I would hope that the Administration keeps that in mind as they seek to replace Mr. Simonson.

There has also been a number of complaints about Administration officials being vague and allusive in their discussions about the types of products they might want to purchase, what quantity, and at what price.

Industry representatives have said that this type of uncertainty is a detriment to the process and has discouraged many companies from participating in the program. The biotech industry would prefer a system more akin to the Department of Defense's countermeasure program, where government purchasing is much more reliable. And I would be interested to hear recommendations from the witnesses about how we can bridge the difference between these two models, even though the populations they are designed to protect vary greatly.

The obvious concern and another complaint is that the program simply does not provide enough incentives for biotech firms to research and develop countermeasures. Industry has said that they need significantly more incentives in order to play in the game. One such proposal, commonly referred to as a wild card extension, would extend the life of a patent for any drug of a company that develops new defenses against biological weapons. This would allow drug makers to extend its patent on its most profitable drugs, even though it may be completely unrelated to a bioterrorism threat. The drug industry claims that extending the patent on blockbuster drugs is needed to encourage firms to make up for the loss they incur by developing less profitable countermeasures, but I could not disagree more with that. Such a proposal simply is another way to provide windfall profits for the pharmaceutical industry and would keep prescription drug prices unnecessarily high, in my opinion.

Furthermore, I would think that enough incentives currently exist for drug manufacturers and biotech companies to enter the market, after my Republican friends provided them with sweeping new liability protections as part of the Defense Authorization Bill for 2006. In fact, last year, in the dead of night, Republicans included a provision that would allow lawsuits against vaccine manufacturers only in the case of willful misconduct, and this is a much higher standard than negligence, which is more commonly used in product liability cases. Furthermore, the Secretary can apply this liability shield to any product used to treat an epidemic or a pandemic, which is left to be defined by the Secretary. If that isn't enough incentive for the drug industry to enter the market, I don't know what is.

And finally, Mr. Chairman, as we examine the success of Project BioShield, I think it is important for us to consider whether or not the funding level we authorized two years ago is adequate to accomplish the goals that we laid out. Congress authorized only $5.6 billion over ten years for Project BioShield and established specific timeframes in which that money could be spent. Incidentally, more than $1 billion of that money has already been obligated to the four contracts currently approved under the program. Accordingly, as we move forward, we may want to consider adding additional funds, especially for greater government investment in research and development.

But again, thank you for calling today's hearing, Mr. Chairman. Clearly, there are some areas of Project BioShield that may need to be fixed for the program to work properly and to that end, I look forward to working with you and the rest of my colleagues on the committee in a bipartisan fashion to meet these goals, the same way we did two years ago, and the health and safety of our citizens deserve, certainly, no less than that. Thank you.

MR. DEAL. I thank the gentleman. Ms. Myrick, do you have an opening statement? All right. Well, we will proceed to our panel, then.

[Additional statements submitted for the record follow:]

PREPARED STATEMENT OF THE HON. JOE BARTON, CHAIRMAN, COMMITTEE ON ENERGY AND COMMERCE

Thank you, Mr. Chairman.

I want to commend you for holding this important hearing. The known threats of the 20th Century have given way to new unforeseen threats we cannot ignore. While there has been no successful attack on our homeland since 9-11, the Committee must diligently oversee and strengthen the components of the U.S. biodefense structure that we helped launch.

The legislative pieces of this biodefense structure include:

- The Public Health and Bioterrorism Preparedness and Response Act;
- The public health provisions of the Homeland Security Act;
- The Small Pox Emergency Personnel Protection Act;
- The Project Bioshield Act;
- Provisions in the Faster and Smarter Funding for First Responders Act; and
- The Public Readiness and Emergency Preparedness Act.

These authorization efforts have been matched by substantial increases in spending by the Department of Health and Human Services, the National Institutes of Health, the Department of Homeland Security, and the Department of Defense. The money goes for research, development and acquisition of medical countermeasures against chemical, biological, radiological and nuclear threats. In fact, Congress recently appropriated billions of dollars to take countermeasures against pandemic flu.

The Energy and Commerce Committee has a strong record of accomplishment in homeland security, including on biodefense. We must continue to develop policies which improve biodefense capabilities. Real risks must be matched with useful and effective countermeasures. We need to ensure these programs are working well together. I look forward to hearing from today's witnesses on the status of Project Bioshield and on ideas for its improvement.

PREPARED STATEMENT OF THE HON. BARBARA CUBIN, A REPRESENTATIVE IN CONGRESS FROM THE STATE OF WYOMING

Thank you Mr. Chairman.

I have always been a national security hawk, something that has taken on new meanings as the American people face emerging threats to their safety and well-being.

By passing the Project Bioshield Act of 2004, Congress recognized the need for countermeasures to chemical, biological, radiological and nuclear threats. While there is no question Project Bioshield has proven useful, questions remain as to how to improve both the law itself, as well as how to facilitate a more cohesive implementation of the law by the various Executive Branch agencies involved.

I hope today's testimony will also call more attention to the threat posed by naturally-occurring infectious diseases. An influenza pandemic, for example, is certainly on par with the threat of bioterrorism in terms of its national security implications. And yet the U.S. currently lacks the vaccine supply and production capacity to mitigate such a pandemic.

That's why myself and Rep. Brian Baird have introduced H.R. 3154, the Infectious Diseases Research and Development Act of 2005. This bipartisan bill would provide the market incentives needed to spur private research and development into infectious disease products, which are simply not as lucrative as the drugs you might see advertised on television.

The threat of bioterrorism is very real, and very dangerous, but we cannot let it overshadow other public health threats that hold the potential for equally devastating consequences.

We will hear calls for more funding today in order to produce a more comprehensive approach under Project Bioshield, though we must face the reality that it would be impossible to stockpile an adequate supply of drugs for each and every bio-threat. I hope our panelists will have suggestions for how we can streamline countermeasure development so we can make them quickly when we need them.

Amidst calls for funding, I would also encourage my colleagues to also consider potential market-based solutions to our drug development problems, such as the ones included in H.R. 3154.

MR. DEAL. I am pleased to introduce the first panel. First is the Honorable Alex M. Azar, Deputy Secretary, U.S. Department of Health and Human Services. Next, Mr. Jean D. Reed, and I am going to have to take a deep breath to read this one, Special Assistant, Chemical and Biological Defense and Chemical Demilitarization Programs, Office of the Assistant to the Secretary of Defense for Nuclear and Chemical and Biological Defense. I don't know what that acronym is, but it has got to be one doozy.

MR. REED. It is unpronounceable, sir.

MR. DEAL. Gentleman, we are pleased to have you here today. Your written statements have been made a part of the record, and we would welcome your oral testimony and hopefully summarize the written portion that you have submitted. We will begin with you, Mr. Azar.

STATEMENTS OF THE ALEX M. AZAR, DEPUTY SECRETARY, U.S. DEPARTMENT OF HEALTH AND HUMAN SERVICES; AND JEAN D. REED, SPECIAL ASSISTANT, CHEMICAL AND BIOLOGICAL DEFENSE AND CHEMICAL DEMILITARIZATION PROGRAMS, OFFICE OF THE ASSISTANT TO THE SECRETARY OF DEFENSE, U.S. DEPARTMENT OF DEFENSE

MR. AZAR. Good afternoon, Mr. Chairman and members of the subcommittee. Thank you very much. I am pleased to be here today to update you on the steps that HHS has been taking to implement the Project BioShield Act.

Many countermeasures for potential agents of terrorism realistically have no market other than the Government and thus have not generated a great deal of manufacturers. Because the market for developing countermeasures is speculative, without government interest private, companies have not invested and engaged in developing the countermeasures that the current situation warrants. Project BioShield was intended to provide such an assurance of a market. I want to acknowledge the important role of this committee in enactment of Project BioShield and thank you for your continued support of this critical program.

The Office of Research Development Coordination within the Office of Public Health and Emergency Preparedness at HHS exercises and coordinates the procurement authorities utilizing the Special Reserve Fund authorized under Project BioShield. Prioritization and development of requirements for medical countermeasures and medical countermeasure acquisition programs is coordinated by the expert interagency Weapons of Mass Destruction Medical Countermeasures Subcommittee, another long name. In setting priorities for medical countermeasure acquisition under Project BioShield, this interagency subcommittee considers a number of factors. The credibility and immediacy of the specific threats are driving factors and are informed by material threat assessments that are conducted by the Department of Homeland Security. Other factors include an evaluation of the availability of appropriate countermeasures, both current and projected, and the target population for which medical countermeasures would be used.

To date, HHS has implemented acquisition programs addressing each of the four threat agents determined to be material threats to the U.S. population by the Department of Homeland Security: anthrax, smallpox, botulinum toxins, and radiological/nuclear agents. HHS has used the special reserved fund to award two contracts for vaccines against anthrax, one contract for a liquid formulation of a drug to protect children from radioactive iodine exposure following nuclear events, and one contract for agents countering the effects of internal exposure to transuranic radioisotopes.

In addition, negotiations are underway currently for the acquisition of anthrax therapeutic antitoxins, and countermeasures to address the blood-related deficiencies associated with acute radiation syndrome. With respect to smallpox vaccines, an award will be made for the manufacture and delivery of up to 20 million doses of a next generation attenuated smallpox vaccine called modified vaccinia Ankara. Additionally, negotiations are underway for procuring 200,000 doses of botulinum antitoxin.

The experience implementing BioShield has highlighted challenges. The potential payoff for a breakthrough in medical countermeasures against chemical, biological, and nuclear/radiological, CBRN threats, is modest when compared with other drugs. For example, the global market for just one cholesterol-lowering agent exceeds the global market for all vaccines together, not just those that comprise a security countermeasure. Additionally, it is estimated that the cost of developing and bringing to market a new drug is between $800 million and $1.7 billion per drug. In addition, for a countermeasure to be eligible for Project BioShield, solid clinical experience and/or research data must support "a reasonable conclusion that the countermeasure will qualify for FDA approval or licensure within eight years after the date of a determination." Only then is the countermeasure eligible for funding from the $5.6 billion Special Reserve Fund. Late stage research and development funds that can support advanced product development of potential BioShield candidates before they are BioShield eligible are therefore critical to ensuring a robust pipeline. To address this, HHS has proposed $160 million for advanced research and development in the fiscal year 2007 budget to support promising candidates while shifting risk away from Project BioShield acquisition programs.

We recognize that more can and must be done to aggressively and efficiently implement Project BioShield. Secretary Leavitt has already announced his intention to establish a dedicated strategic planning function in HHS that more efficiently integrates biodefense requirements across the full range of threat agents, with the execution of advanced development and procurement of medical countermeasures. He will assign and empower the Office of Public Health Emergency Preparedness as the responsible office to develop and implement a strategic plan for this purpose, and will ensure that HHS component programs and functions are properly aligned and that their respect strengths are leveraged to support the Office of Public Health Emergency Preparedness' efforts. We will also work to streamline and make more effective the current BioShield interagency governance process. We will make this process more transparent and work to educate the public and industry about our priorities and opportunities. As part of this, HHS will convene an outreach meeting with external stakeholders later this year.

During the first 20 months of Project BioShield, HHS has used this legislation to initiate major acquisition programs for medical countermeasures to biological and radiological/nuclear threats, to expedite the award of grants and contracts for research to identify and develop medical countermeasures to protect the U.S. population from chemical, biological, radiological, and nuclear threat agents, and to provide access to the best available medical countermeasures in emergency situations.

Mr. Chairman, thank you once again for inviting me to testify on our efforts and to update you on the Department's plans for the future, and at the appropriate time, I would be happy to take any questions.

[The prepared statement of the Hon. Alex M. Azar follows:]

PREPARED STATEMENT OF THE HONORABLE ALEX M. AZAR, DEPUTY SECRETARY, U.S. DEPARTMENT OF HEALTH AND HUMANS SERVICES

Good afternoon Chairman Deal and Members of the Subcommittee. I am pleased to be here today to update you on the steps the Department of Health and Human Services (HHS) has taken to implement the Project BioShield Act of 2004 (P.L.108-276). Project Bioshield, as announced by President Bush in his State of the Union address on January 28, 2003, was proposed to accelerate the process of research, development, purchase, and availability of effective countermeasures against agents of bioterror. Then HHS Secretary Tommy Thompson and Department of Homeland Security (DHS) Secretary Tom Ridge jointly transmitted the "Project BioShield Act of 2003" to Congress on February 26, 2003 and it was signed into law by President Bush on July 21, 2004.

Project BioShield enables the Government to develop, procure, and make available countermeasures to chemical, biological, radiological, and nuclear agents for use in a public health emergency that affects national security. Pharmaceutical research and development historically has focused on development of products likely to attract significant commercial interest. Many countermeasures for potential agents of terrorism realistically have no market other than the government and thus have not generated a great deal of manufacturer interest. Because the market for developing countermeasures is speculative, without government interest, private companies have not invested and engaged in developing the countermeasures that the current situation warrants. Project BioShield was intended to provide such an assurance of a market. I want to acknowledge the important role of this Committee in enactment of Project BioShield and thank you for your continued support of the program.

Project BioShield is a critical part of a broader strategy to defend America against the threat of weapons of mass destruction. It provides HHS with several new authorities to speed the research, development, acquisition, and availability of medical countermeasures to defend against chemical, biological, radiological and nuclear (CBRN) threats. Defending against such threats is a top priority for the Bush Administration and having an appropriate armamentarium of medical countermeasures is a critical element of the response and recovery component of the President's "21st Century Strategy for Biodefense." HHS acts to accomplish this mission through integrated efforts of several components, including: research and development at the National Institutes of Health (NIH); regulatory activities related to medical countermeasure development and availability at the Food and Drug Administration (FDA); acquisition of medical countermeasures through the Office of Public Health Emergency Preparedness (OPHEP); and storage and deployment in an emergency by the Centers for Disease Control and Prevention.

NIH BioShield Authorities

HHS's National Institutes of Health (NIH) is assigned the lead role in the research and early development of medical countermeasures to prepare for and respond to CBRN agents and in the conduct of research to expand our understanding of the human health impact of these agents. The National Institute of Allergy and Infectious Diseases (NIAID) is the NIH institute with primary responsibility for carrying out this assignment. Thus far, NIAID has used Project BioShield authorities to award $35.6 million in grants and contracts. These awards will promote development of countermeasures toward possible future procurement with Project BioShield funds. Twelve grants and two contracts have been awarded to support research directed against the Category A agents that cause anthrax, smallpox, tularemia, plague, botulism, and viral hemorrhagic fevers. NIAID has awarded 4 grants and 3 contracts to support research on medical countermeasures against radiological or nuclear terrorist attacks, including countermeasures to protect the immune system against radiation and improved treatments for the elimination of internal radionuclide contamination that can be given by mouth rather than intravenously.

Medical Countermeasure Acquisition

The Office of Research and Development Coordination (ORDC) within OPHEP exercises and coordinates the procurement authorities utilizing the Special Reserve Fund authorized under Project BioShield. ORDC works with NIH, CDC, and FDA to coordinate the transitions between medical countermeasures development at NIH, procurement by ORDC, storage and development by CDC, and approval/licensure/clearance by FDA. Prioritization and development of requirements for medical countermeasures acquisition programs is coordinated by the Weapons of Mass Destruction Medical Countermeasures (WMD MCM) Subcommittee. By defining requirements for medical countermeasures the Subcommittee enables policy makers to identify and evaluate acquisition options to address immediate and future needs.

In setting priorities for medical countermeasure acquisition under Project BioShield, the WMD MCM Subcommittee considers a number of factors. The credibility and immediacy of the specific threats are driving factors and are informed by Material Threat Assessments (MTAs) conducted by the DHS. Other factors include an evaluation of the availability of appropriate countermeasures, both current and projected, and the target population for which the medical countermeasure would be used. In addition, logistical issues are considered such as the feasibility of deployment in a public health emergency, shelf life, and the storage and maintenance requirements.

To date the WMD MCM Subcommittee has defined USG requirements and acquisition options for eight medical countermeasures. These HHS acquisition programs address each of the four threat agents determined to be Material Threats to the U.S. population by DHS [*Bacillus anthracis* (anthrax), smallpox virus, botulinum toxins, and radiological/nuclear agents]. Such agents are determined to present a material threat to the U.S. sufficient to affect national security. HHS has used the Special Reserve Fund (SRF) to award two contracts for vaccines against anthrax, one contract for a liquid formulation of a drug to protect children from radioactive iodine exposure following nuclear events, and one contract for chelating agents for countering the effects of internal exposure to transuranic radioisotopes.

In addition, negotiations are underway for the acquisition of anthrax therapeutics, and countermeasures to address the blood-related deficiencies associated with acute radiation syndrome. With respect to smallpox vaccines, an award will be made for the manufacture and delivery of up to 20 million doses of a next generation attenuated smallpox vaccine, modified vaccinia Ankara (MVA). Additionally, negotiations are underway for procuring 200,000 doses of botulinum antitoxin.

These countermeasures are being added to the Strategic National Stockpile (SNS) that currently includes vaccines, antibiotics to counter infections caused by anthrax and plague, antitoxins, chemical antidotes and radiation emergency medical countermeasures.

Emergency Use Authorization

Project BioShield thus provides an important tool for the acquisition of safe and effective medical countermeasures, licensed or approved by the FDA for addressing CBRN threat agents. BioShield also recognized however that, should CBRN agents threaten the U.S. before these countermeasures are procured, the American people should be provided access to the best available alternatives. These could include products that are FDA-approved for a different use or those that have not yet obtained FDA-approval, but for which sufficient safety and efficacy data is available to support their emergency use.

The HHS Secretary delegated the authority to issue "Emergency Use Authorizations" (EUAs) to the FDA Commissioner and to date FDA has issued one EUA. The Deputy Secretary of Defense determined in December 2004 that there was a significant potential for a military emergency involving a heightened risk to U.S. military forces of attack with anthrax. Based on this determination, then-Secretary Thompson declared an emergency justifying the authorization of the emergency use of anthrax vaccine and in January 2005, the FDA authorized the emergency use of the licensed Anthrax Vaccine Adsorbed (AVA) for the prevention of inhalation anthrax for individuals between 18 and 65 years of age who are deemed by the DOD to be at heightened risk of exposure due to attack with anthrax. As conditions of this authorization, each potential AVA recipient was informed of the benefits and risks of this emergency use of AVA and of their option to refuse or accept AVA administration. The authorization for this emergency use of AVA ended one year from the declaration of the emergency in January 2006.

Strategic National Stockpile

Medical countermeasure availability also requires well-planned stockpile and deployment strategies, and all acquisitions made under Project BioShield include close consultations with the CDC to ensure these medicines will be rapidly available if needed. CDC operates HHS's Strategic National Stockpile (SNS), which contains large quantities of medicine and medical supplies to protect the American public if there is a public health emergency severe enough to cause local supplies to be inadequate. Once Federal and local authorities agree that the SNS is needed, medicines and medical supplies can be delivered to any State in the U.S. within 12 hours. Consequently, each State is now required to develop plans to receive and distribute SNS medicine and medical supplies to local communities as quickly as possible in the event of a deployment.

Challenges to Implementation

The experience implementing BioShield over the past 21 months has highlighted a number of issues that make acquisitions under Project BioShield challenging and unique.

For example, while liability issues have not prevented the completion of any countermeasure acquisitions to date, liability protection remains a major source of concern to industry, and a recurring theme in the Project BioShield acquisition process. Therefore, we are pleased that Congress last year passed the "Public Readiness and Emergency Preparedness (PREP) Act" as part of the 2006 Defense Appropriations Act (P.L. 109-148). This legislation included liability protections for manufacturers of security and pandemic countermeasures. We believe this will further create industry interest and progress in this area.

Project BioShield acquisitions have also not drawn the attention of large pharmaceutical or biotechnology firms. The potential payoff for a breakthrough in medical countermeasures against CBRN threats is modest when compared with other drugs. For example, the global market for just one cholesterol-lowering agent exceeds the global market for *all* vaccines together, not just those that comprise a security countermeasure. Additionally, it is estimated that the cost of developing and bringing to market a new drug is between $800 million and $1.7 billion.

Smaller companies have been attracted to participate in Project BioShield, which results in an expansion of pharmaceutical manufacturing capacity and expertise. A cost to building this capacity among smaller, less experienced companies, however, requires more intensive technical assistance. Unlike the larger, more experienced pharmaceutical firms, these smaller companies require increased levels of federal government assistance and oversight to meet the requirements of Project BioShield procurement contracts and mitigate the risk of failure. HHS has demonstrated a successful track record of enhancing the infrastructure of smaller, less established biotechnology firms, as evidenced by the HHS acquisition programs completed before Project BioShield. Continued successes will require a sustained commitment of federal resources to ensure proper contract oversight and administration, and to ensure that such less-established contractors meet their regulatory and production milestones as may be contractually required.

Notwithstanding limited Secretarial authority to make payments up to 10 percent of the contract cost, the Project BioShield Act of 2004 provides "that no payment shall be made until delivery has been made of a portion, acceptable to the Secretary, of the total number of units contracted for." This requirement constitutes a significant risk for small biotechnology firms, in particular, that may not have the necessary financial resources available to support final advanced product development prior to receipt of payment.

Finally, for a countermeasure to be eligible for Project BioShield, solid clinical experience and/or research data must support "a reasonable conclusion that the countermeasure will qualify for [FDA] approval or licensure within eight years after the date of a determination." Only then is the countermeasure eligible for funding from the $5.6 billion Special Reserve Fund. Late stage research and development funds that can support advanced product development of potential BioShield candidates before they are BioShield eligible are therefore critical to ensuring a robust pipeline. To address this, HHS has proposed $160 M for advanced development in the FY07 budget to support promising candidates while shifting risk away from Project BioShield acquisition programs.

Future Plans

We recognize that more can and must be done to aggressively and efficiently implement Project BioShield. Secretary Leavitt has announced his intention to establish a dedicated strategic planning function in HHS that more efficiently integrates biodefense requirements, across the full range of threat agents, with the execution of advanced development and procurement of medical countermeasures. HHS will assign and empower the Office of Public Health Emergency Preparedness (OPHEP) as the responsible office to develop and implement a strategic plan for this purpose, and will ensure that HHS component programs and functions are properly aligned, and that their respective strengths are leveraged, to support OPHEP's efforts. We will also work closely with other departments and agencies to streamline and make more effective the current BioShield interagency governance process. We will make this process more transparent and work to educate the public and industry about our priorities and opportunities. As part of this, HHS will convene an outreach meeting with these external stakeholders later this year.

As we move forward, we would also like to thank Members of Congress for their interest in improving the BioShield program, and we look forward to continuing to work with you.

Conclusions

During the first 21 months of Project BioShield, HHS has used the provisions of this legislation to initiate major acquisition programs for medical countermeasures to biological and radiological/nuclear threats, to expedite the award of grants and contracts for research to identify and develop medical countermeasures to protect the U.S. population from chemical, biological, radiological, and nuclear threat agents, and to provide access to the best available medical countermeasures in emergency situations.

Thank you once again for inviting me to testify on our efforts and update you on the Department's plans for the future.

I would be happy to take any questions.

MR. DEAL. Thank you. Mr. Reed?

MR. REED. Mr. Chairman, thank you very much for inviting me to appear before the committee today. I am, as you have already indicated, the Special Assistant for Chemical and Biological Defense and Chemical Demilitarization Programs. No, it is not pronounceable as an acronym. The office is essentially that of the Deputy Assistant to the Secretary of Defense for Nuclear and Chemical and Biological programs. In that area, I support Dr. Dale Klein, who is the Assistant to the Secretary of Defense for Nuclear and Chemical and Biological, and the office was established in the early 1990s by Congress to centralize and provide a focal point for the Chemical and Biological Defense Program within the Department of Defense. I have been on the job for about three months. I came to that job from 15 years as a professional staffer for the House Armed Services Committee. In that role, I had the enjoyable task of working with your staff in the development of the Defense BioShield Act of 2003 and then working in concert with them on BioShield Act of 2004, and I found that an exceedingly rewarding experience. You have a very dedicated staff on that, and sir, I give my compliments. It has been delightful to work with them, although we, at times, had differing views on certain issues.

Nevertheless, I find myself today in this position on the other side of the table, faced with a very challenging position as we prepare U.S. forces for both action on the battlefield and being prepared to operate in a potentially contaminated environment, contaminated by chemical and biological agents, and also from the standpoint from the ability of that force to operate in support of homeland defense and homeland security.

The Assistant to the Secretary of Defense for NCB programs, as I indicated, serves as the focal point for overseeing the Department's chemical and biological defense research, development, and acquisition. In preparation of the fiscal year 2007 President's budget submission of approximately $1.5 billion for this program, a process was used which ensures that the Department's efforts in CBRN, chemical, biological, radiological, and nuclear defense, are closely aligned with strategic guidance and are driven by operational requirements rather than being driven specifically by technological approaches. A major aspect of the planning phase, following from the National Military Strategy and the National Security Strategy, is a joint capabilities development process. That approach to planning serves to focus attention on the requirement capabilities, while providing guidance to fit programs within the resources available, and to meet defense goals. A top priority is given to dissuading, deterring, and defeating those who seek to harm the United States directly, including those extremist individuals or organizations that may possess and employ weapons of mass destruction.

The current strategy emphasizes a capabilities-based approach rather than the approach in the past, which provided greater emphasis on prioritizing threat agents and targeting budgetary resources based on validated intelligence. You may remember that the law was changed a couple of years ago to get away from the fact that we could only focus the Chemical and Biological Defense Program against validated threat agents. Because of the developments in medical technology, the potential threat posed by bioengineered threats, that law was widened to permit the program to concentrate on almost anything that could be out there, but to do it in a very measured manner.

Key capabilities within the Chemical and Biological Defense Program are structured within the operational elements of sense. That is, remote sensing standoff detection and identification systems; shape, battle space management, including modeling and simulation and the communication and decision systems that enable the commander to make appropriate responses and plans; shield, collective, and individual protection and preventative medicines, such as vaccine; and sustain capabilities for decontamination and medical diagnostics and therapeutics. As a supplement to this joint capabilities development process, the Secretary of Defense has provided direction to enhance the overall chemical and biological defense posture. A major element coming out of the Quadrennial Defense Review is the establishment of a program called Green Line, nickname, or Transformational Medical Technology Initiative, that is aimed specifically at attacking the threat of bioengineered diseases, bioengineered agents. Approximately $1.5 billion over the future years defense plan has been allocated to that. That program is in source selection at this point and is being closely coordinated with what is going on within Health and Human Services and Homeland Security, and we will be able to say more about that in detail after the source selection process is completed in about another month or so.

It is a challenging program that faces us. It is closely coordinated with the efforts of the Departments of Health and Human Services and with the Department of Homeland Security, and it also does address what is going on in the BioShield Program. One of the features of the defense BioShield legislation, when we did that in 2003, was to emphasize to the Secretary of Defense the necessity of coordinating closely with Health and Human Services and with Homeland Security in the development of the overall research and development programs and acquisition programs so in fact the Department of Defense would be able to leverage their efforts and vice versa. That work is ongoing. We can get into that in the question and answer period, if you so desire. And it is again a pleasure to be here and I look forward to your questions.

MR. DEAL. I thank you. We will start the questioning at this time. Mr. Azar, I understand that under Project BioShield, the Department of Homeland Security has a role in determining material threats and the Department of Defense has its own program, that has just been outlined by Mr. Reed, to address chemical, biological, radiological and nuclear threats. But it seems to me that HHS has the most expertise with respect to medical and health issues and emerging threats, the Department of Homeland Security has expertise on terrorism as a threat. Would you explain to us how these responsibilities have been working? And would it make more sense if HHS was allowed to determine the medical aspects of what constitutes a material threat, and how does DOD threat assessment process work in relation to the material threat process?

MR. AZAR. Thank you, Mr. Chairman. In terms of the Department of Homeland Security's material threat assessment and determination process, they play a very critical role in this process. We at HHS, we know health, but we don't know the threats that our Nation faces. We aren't an intelligence agency, and what DHS has the ability to do is to pull together all the strands of information in the intelligence community and assess across the broad spectrum the threats and help prioritize them for making those material threat assessments and determinations. We certainly assist them in that process by providing our health expertise. They have their own, but we also provide that, as do the health experts within the intelligence community. So I am quite satisfied that the health expertise input happens and gets into that process. But it is important for an agency like DHS, that has the ability to pull all of the different strands of intelligence into it and compare threats, to make those material threat determinations. And then we, of course, under the Project BioShield statute, Secretary Leavitt have to also make a determination that the acquisition is necessary for the public health. And so this gets coordinated also through these interagency weapons of mass destruction subcommittee. That is where really a highly technical qualified expert body of individuals drives the engine of this process.

MR. DEAL. Mr. Reed, do you agree and would you comment further on that coordination?

MR. REED. If I may. As it happens, and it wasn't done with a forethought with respect to today's hearing, but coming out of the meetings of the Weapons of Mass Destruction Medical Countermeasures Subcommittee last week, was a meeting at the action officer level of Department of Defense Health Affairs, my office, the Department of Health and Human Services, and the Department of Homeland Security, to address specifically this area. You know, coming back into the Department, even though I watched the program very closely from my vantage point on the House Armed Services Committee, to look afresh at the overall threat to our military forces.

But now, in the broader context of homeland security as well, we met with the Defense Intelligence Agency, began to discuss the sorts of issues that needed to be looked at in terms of near-term threats and a near-term assessment of that, extending on perhaps to something as long term, a year, perhaps a year-plus, of development of a new national intelligence estimate on the part of the DIA. Now that will need to be something that represents the entire intelligence community as it comes forward, and we are just making, really, the first steps in that, to begin to update what is there right now. The threat is changing, there is no question about that, and we need to have our eyes open as we approach that.

MR. DEAL. Mr. Azar, under Project BioShield, the Secretary of the Department of Homeland Security, in consultation with the Secretary of HHS, is charged with assessing current and emerging threats of chemical, biological, radiological, and nuclear agents, and determines which of these agents present a material threat against the United States population sufficient to affect national security. What I would like to know, because we have had a lot of testimony on this issue, is if the H5N1 virus, or pandemic flu in general, fits under this definition, and if it doesn't, would you explain why it doesn't?

MR. AZAR. Mr. Chairman, as you know, $5.6 billion is in the Special Reserve Fund for Project BioShield, and that is a lot of money. But in the scheme of developing medical countermeasures and drugs and devices that would be used for chemical, biological, radiological, and nuclear incidents, it is not an infinite supply of money. That is why this threat analysis that has to occur by DHS becomes so important that it is intentional, that if we expand beyond intentional threats, those harms, we could rapidly dissipate that limited amount of money that we need for the very real intentional threats against our country out of that. Now, when it has come to issues like pandemic influenza, we thank you and other Members of Congress for the strong support you have given when we have had naturally occurring threats. Coming to Congress and working with you to get the first year of the President's requested funding on pandemic avian influenza to respond to that threat, as you know, that only, pandemic influenza preparedness alone would have evacuated the Special Reserve Fund here, just as one example. So I think both are critical, but I do think it is important to keep, in this context of BioShield acquisition, those two separate. Now, if we talk advanced research and development, certainly there is an important role that we ought to be playing, and I think we ought to be doing a better job of supporting advanced R and D for both the intentional threats and the naturally occurring threats.

MR. DEAL. I take it that the policy answer is that it does not fit the definition. Could I ask you, if you would, to have legal counsel within HHS to answer the question as to whether it meets the legal definition or not?

MR. AZAR. Yes, sir, absolutely. We will get back to you on that.

MR. DEAL. Okay. And my time is expired. Mr. Pallone.

MR. PALLONE. Thank you, Mr. Chairman. Mr. Azar, I wanted to ask you some questions about this liability language and then also about the wild card patent extension. As you know, the fiscal year 2006 DOD appropriations conference report contained liability language that was not part of either the House or Senate-passed appropriation bills. But first, I would like to know if you or anyone in your department was involved in drafting or reviewing or providing technical assistance, policy advice, or in any other way was involved in the development of the language that found itself in that DOD appropriations conference report.

MR. AZAR. Congressman, yes, we were involved in providing technical assistance on the drafting of that and trying to provide the best advice. This is a process driven by Congress, but it was something the President had asked for, and said that as part of pandemic influenza preparedness, a critical element of being able to get manufacturers to produce the products that we need was removing the liability barrier. So this was very much a centerpiece, a sine qua non of moving towards pandemic preparedness.

MR. PALLONE. All right. Then, in the same line, I mean, obviously, you are familiar with the liability language. Can you provide us with your views on the substantive merits of that language in the conference report and specifically, does it, in your view, take complete care of all legitimate liability concerns of the Administration, in terms of attracting private sector participation in BioShield, or do you think further changes are either necessary or desirable?

MR. AZAR. As we were working on developing the pandemic plan, the President's plan, he, the Secretary, and others met with those who we needed to work with on developing the type of countermeasures, the vaccines, the antivirals, in this area and the vaccine industry came to us and it was quite clear, in our own experience demonstrated this, that there were several barriers, one of which was liability. And we believe that the language that was produced here should remove the hurdle of liability in terms of moving forward here. Obviously, industry will end up providing its perspective, but we believe that this should resolve the liability concerns that we had heard about in the process, and plan to be moving forward on the pandemic acquisitions on that basis.

MR. PALLONE. Now, what about whether or not you think any further changes are necessary or desirable to attract private sector participation in BioShield, beyond the liability provision?

MR. AZAR. Well, on the separate issue of BioShield, we do believe that some of the proposals that are currently being put forward, Senator Burr has been very active on the Senate side with a package of legislation that really goes in the right direction in terms of focusing attention this period on advanced research and development. There is the earlier stage of basis primary research that NIH does, and then there is Project BioShield, which is about acquiring products that are already ready to put into the stockpile. But there is this hurdle between those two, of advanced research and development, where we do believe there needs to be this type of collaborative working with industry, incubating that along, providing funding in partnership with industry to remove some of the risk of the very risky development. That is why we have requested the $160 million in the 2007 budget for that, and that is why part of the pandemic plan has significant advanced R and D funding on, for instance, agetent research, next generation antivirals, on advanced R and D to deal with that interim period.

MR. PALLONE. Well, let me just ask one other thing. You know, the liability language only mentions compensation for persons who are injured by a covered countermeasure. Do you have any intention to submit any kind of legislative language for a compensation program? I mean, would you support some sort of compensation program for people who are injured?

MR. AZAR. The hurdle and the issue that we were trying to, and had to, overcome to be able to move forward and make the money that Congress appropriated useful was the liability concern, getting the manufacturers to actually be willing to produce the products, to test the products and allow us to acquire them. Compensation is an issue that, as we move along, we would be happy to work with Congress on and talk about. It is not the hurdle towards the development and--

MR. PALLONE. But you don't have a specific compensation program that you are thinking about or funding for at this point?

MR. AZAR. No, sir.

MR. PALLONE. Okay. I wanted to ask about the wild card patent extension. I only have a couple of minutes here, Mr. Chairman. You know, I am concerned, as I said before, about providing incentives at the expense of the American public and U.S. health care. I mean, I think this is the type of thing that the pharmaceuticals industry could simply take advantage of. So I guess my question really would be do you want to comment on that at all, on this wild-card patent extension? I mean I am obviously critical of it. I think that it has the potential to just provide, you know, some kind of windfall for the industry.

MR. AZAR. We do not have any views established on the issue of this wild card separately. We do agree with you, as you said in your opening statement, that we do need to focus on the incentives for getting businesses into the Project BioShield CBRN countermeasures industry. It is a very risky industry. We are the only purchaser for most of these products. It is an uncertain market, and that is why a lot of what we want to do is make ourselves a better business partner as we move forward on implementing Project BioShield, in terms of transparency, in terms of predictability. We really want to move that focus forward and so that is where the focus of--

MR. PALLONE. You don't have a position on that?

MR. AZAR. No, we don't.

MR. PALLONE. All right, thank you, Mr. Chairman, for the extra time.

MR. DEAL. You are welcome. Ms. Myrick, you are recognized for questions.

MS. MYRICK. You asked the question I had.

MR. DEAL. All right. Mr. Shimkus is next.

MR. SHIMKUS. Thank you, Mr. Chairman. Secretary Azar, we seem to have two camps with separate priorities on how money should be spent on this issue. Some believe we should spend money procuring vaccines that are readily available, and the others believe we should spend money to develop future vaccines. How do we bridge the gap on this conflict and what is the Administration's priority?

MR. AZAR. Congressman, thank you for that question. It is a difficult issue and this is where this relying on the scientific experts and technical experts that are out there, whether it is the Institute of Medicine providing advice or the Interagency Subcommittee of Medical Countermeasures, that brings together the real technical experts from the Defense Department, from the Office of Science Technology Policy, from DHS, from HHS. That is where, frankly, we need to rely on the scientists to decide and to provide us with the recommendations. Is current technology good enough on a certain product, or are we at the time where we need to start pushing forward in developing that next generation technology? And so these are not easy issues. They are science-based, they are technical issues, and that is why getting as much input as we can, I think, is very critical.

MR. SHIMKUS. From the public policy arena, and just following up, obviously, this is real appropriated dollars, real money. And then, in the event of an attack, if we are not prepared, here is the dilemma: we either have the vaccines or we don't. The public is not going to understand our decision not to have readily accessible vaccines, when we say, well, we were preparing for the next case down the line. I am not sure if I should let you off the hook that easy. I mean, we are looking for some help in reconciling this and, Mr. Chairman, I don't know what the answer is.

MR. AZAR. Congressman, sometimes, depending on the nature of the product, some vaccines are pre-event and it would depend on the nature of the threat assessment of an event occurring and the populations that would be hit by it in terms of what size, for instance, you might need to have in your stockpile. Other vaccines, perhaps, could be of assistance in a post-exposure context and it would depend on the product and whether there has been clinical evidence, scientific studies, and FDA approval of post-exposure administration of certain vaccines, whether they might be beneficial.

MR. SHIMKUS. And if I may, prior to shelf life, too? Probably some of these might expire. You buy a whole bunch and nothing happens and they you throw it out.

MR. AZAR. Right. And as we mentioned earlier, $5.6 billion is a lot of money, but it is not indefinite amount of money and so it does require a balance between current acquisitions and new acquisitions. And the core, at least my understanding of Project BioShield, is to not just acquire for the stockpile. We have the strategic national stockpile for buying products, generally, already on the market. One of the core purposes of Project BioShield was really to incent, drive, and build the markets for those next generation countermeasures, and I do think it is important, as we implement that, to keep our eye on that ball of incenting and building those markets as the only purchaser or they will never develop.

MR. SHIMKUS. Well, let me move to Mr. Reed. Mr. Reed, when you contract with private entities to develop products, how are issues of liability and ultimate purchase of those products usually handled?

MR. REED. Congressman, the DOD does provide indemnification for liability issues related to immunization of military personnel, and with respect to the relationship with industry, those are normally negotiated as a part of the contract. I would like to provide, however, a reply for the record on that, because we are three months on board and about a half an inch deep in this area right now.

MR. SHIMKUS. I am sure the Chairman would appreciate seeing that, so we will readily accept it.

MR. REED. Yes, we will.

MR. SHIMKUS. And, Mr. Chairman, that is all I have right now. I yield back.

MR. DEAL. I thank the gentleman. Ms. Eshoo, you are recognized.

MS. ESHOO. Thank you, Mr. Chairman, first of all, for holding this important hearing on the process of reexamining bioterrorism and public health security, and a warm welcome to the panelists today and thank you for your public service. I am sorry I wasn't here to make my opening statement which, of course, will be placed in the record. I also want to recognize that a very distinguished constituent of mine is going to be testifying on the next panel, Bruce Cohen, and he is the CEO of Cellerant Therapeutics. I am very pleased and grateful that he would come across the country to share with us his views today, and thank you, Mr. Chairman, for allowing him to testify.

Let me ask this. I want to echo some of the concerns that Congressman Shimkus just touched on in his time with you. Now, it is my understanding that what the Congress appropriated in 2002, $5.6 billion, correct?

MR. AZAR. Yes, ma'am.

MS. ESHOO. Correct. How much do we have left now of the 5.6.

MR. AZAR. We have obligated about $1.089 billion so far out of that fund.

MS. ESHOO. All right. Well, I think the most important issue with BioShield, I mean, there are so many facets to this, so I don't want to give short shrift to anything or diminish in any way, shape or form, but I think the most important issue, relative to the criticisms of BioShield, is whether we are doing all we can to develop the countermeasures as quickly as we can. And how do you step up to that, either, what is perceived or real in terms of the concern, and what can we do to improve it? This is no doubt, no doubt in my mind, and I think in the entirety of the Congress and the American people would chime in, that the threat of a terrorist attack, whether it is biological or chemical or nuclear weapons, I mean, God help us all, and our top responsibility is to secure the American people. So while $5.6 billion is something that I don't think any of us will ever have in our checking accounts, it was a good start in terms of a very serious commitment of the Congress to address this. So maybe you can both enlighten all of us about where we are right now.

MR. AZAR. Congresswoman, I think you are right. We have made great progress so far in the first 20 months of implementing BioShield. We have had four material threat assessment determinations; anthrax, smallpox, botulinum toxin, and radiological/nuclear agents, that we have been dealing with. We have had eight procurement processes underway, but there is much more that we can do to make this process more efficient, faster and better for--

MS. ESHOO. So when you say that the procurements have been made, this is what is presently stockpiled?

MR. AZAR. There are four procurements that have been made. Some are in process of delivery. Some have been delivered into the stockpile. Some are being made. And then we have open procurements right now that are still pending decision.

MS. ESHOO. Of the procurements that have been made, what percentage is stockpiled?

MR. AZAR. If I could just go through the ones that have been made in terms of the stockpile, the anthrax vaccine absorbed, the first of the five million doses has been delivered to the stockpile. The pediatric potassium iodide, the first 1.7 million one-ounce bottles, has been delivered to the stockpile. And then on the--

MS. ESHOO. Is that the entire order?

MR. AZAR. There has been a contract option exercised in February of 2006 for additional pediatric liquid potassium iodide and that is still pending delivery. And then we have the chelating agent DTPA, a radiological/nuclear product and that, to my understanding has been delivered. That is correct, I am told. But we need to speed up this process. What we need to do in terms of our efforts is first, we have got to develop a broad strategic plan here on moving forward. Instead of individual material threat assessments--

MS. ESHOO. So this is not part of our plan?

MR. AZAR. No, these are, in a sense, low hanging fruit assessments, in that we know these are threats, but what we need to do is an integrated strategic plan that pulls together the broad range of threats. And we need to do this in as transparent a way as possible. For that reason, later this year, we are going to convene all stakeholders in this, and as the process of developing an integrated strategic plan on using the rest of the money--

MS. ESHOO. Well, what I am a little disappointed in, with all due respect, is that these dollars were appropriated in 2004, as I understand it.

MR. AZAR. I believe 2004, ma'am.

MS. ESHOO. All right. Well, you know, there is an important nexus, at least in my view, and I think others, probably yours, that scientific discoveries and the dollars that drive them are twins. I mean, it is an explicable set of bookends. And what I am concerned about is you have spoken to the low-hanging fruit, that is important, and there has to be an important timeframe around all of this when the dollars get out there in order to push the discoveries that are needed that will then find their way to the stockpile. And I think that that is something that we need to have more knowledge about. Is this what your plan is being directed toward, and do you have in mind what percent of this budget you are going to dedicate to that?

MR. AZAR. The idea on doing a strategic plan like this that is public is that it will also streamline the procurement process. If you can front load as much of the decision making about that we ought to procure certain products, that they fit into the strategic plan, and you make that public, it creates greater predictability for industry about the areas that we are going in and the types of quantities that we are looking at so that we can be a better business partner with them and then streamline this interagency process and decision making. So I think this is all very important and constructive.

MS. ESHOO. But when do you anticipate this plan, not only to begin, but do you have a timeframe for it that you anticipate when the plan will be done?

MR. AZAR. We are beginning, obviously, it is not beginning now, but this has been getting worked on. Later this year is when we will have the public engagement with it to make sure that we aren't missing things in the plan, that the stakeholders are bought into it, then sometime soon thereafter is when it would be finalized.

MR. DEAL. The gentlelady's time has expired.

MS. ESHOO. Thank you, Mr. Chairman.

MR. DEAL. Dr. Burgess, you are recognized for questions.

MR. BURGESS. Thank you, Mr. Chairman. Secretary Azar, in response to one of Mr. Pallone's questions about liability, you spoke about the industry's response to liability protection. Can you expound on that just a little bit? How has industry responded to the fact that some liability protection has been built into the legislative language? Do we need to do more? Are there areas in the rulemaking process that are going to need attention? Where are we with that? Is industry comfortable with what we have done?

MR. AZAR. My understanding from what I have been hearing from industry and from the process is that, yes, they are comfortable with what has been done. We have obviously not yet exercised the prep act liability protections in our procurements. We will be moving forward clearly in the context of the pandemic implementation of doing that, but I have not personally heard any concerns that the liability protections that were implemented by Congress are not adequate. We are working forward on the regulatory development process. Congress commissioned us to do some definitional work with the Justice Department and that process is moving forward on just laying out that architecture.

MR. BURGESS. Is that regarding things like potential antitrust violations if industry talks amongst itself?

MR. AZAR. If I remember correctly, that is about providing some definitions of the willful misconduct exception, laying out and fleshing out what that exception is.

MR. BURGESS. To follow up on what Ms. Eshoo was asking you, do you think we are doing a good job of providing that platform of predictability for industry from all areas, from a liability standpoint, from a regulatory standpoint? Is private industry going to be our partner in this?

MR. AZAR. Well, that is our goal and I think that the liability protections were a major advance. I believe the administrative changes that we are working towards in terms of a transparent strategic plan up front are a major, major move forward. I believe that the effort of the Administration and of some of the work in Congress towards funding and pushing towards advanced research and development will really enhance that concept of us working in partnership on developing these products and helping to remove some of the scientific and business risk on developing these types of products, also.

MR. BURGESS. And when can we in Congress and we on this committee, expect to hear about some of the comfort with scientific and business risk so that we can be comforted and in turn project that feeling of confidence to our constituents?

MR. AZAR. Well, I think some of it is the $160 million that is in the President's fiscal year 2007 budget for this advanced research and development, getting that passed and start to implement. That will be a critical step. We have the money on pandemic influenza advanced research and development that we are moving forward on implementing. And so I think, in the pandemic influenza context, we should very soon start to get the feedback on is this type of advanced research and development approach. And so I think it is going to be an iterative process over the next several months of learning from the feedback, is this working, and is this providing the right incentives.

MR. BURGESS. Well, I would point that Mr. Shimkus correctly pointed out that the public doesn't have yet general confidence, and doesn't understand why we don't have protection from the pandemic flu. And I would further submit that the public doesn't understand why they don't have protection from the regular seasonal flu every year, from which 15,000 to 30,000 people die. So it is a real concern out there amongst the people we represent, and I will just tell you that it is a real concern of mine here in Congress. I guess one of the other things, and I don't know whether this falls under your jurisdiction or not, but what about the distributive networks that are out there in the event of a pandemic. How comfortable do you feel about where we are with developing those things?

MR. AZAR. We still have a long way to go on ensuring that State and local distribution plans really will line up. The Secretary and I have been traveling around to all 50 States with the Governors hosting the pandemic flu summits. And one of the key messages there is, we can have everything in the stockpile, but it is not going to do any good if it can't effectively be distributed. This is an area where the Federal government has a role, but the dominant role on distributing pharmaceuticals or vaccines is going to be through the State and local arenas, and we are working with them on plans. We have the Cities Readiness Initiative that this committee has been very involved in to enhance the capability in the larger cities of how do you get drugs and vaccines to people in the right period of time. So this remains a major challenge, is the distribution.

MR. BURGESS. Sure, and Mr. Shimkus just pointed out to me that it would be a major concern if it were eliminated in, say, a devastating event such as a Katrina or an earthquake. For that reason, I would just point out that north-central Texas is very stable. We have no hurricanes. We have no earthquakes. Occasional dust storms. I will yield back, Mr. Chairman.

MR. DEAL. I thank the gentleman. Ms. Cubin, you are recognized for questions.

MRS. CUBIN. Thank you, Mr. Chairman. I also want to thank you for calling this hearing today. I would like to start by questioning Deputy Secretary Azar. Does the Administration's BioShield portfolio include naturally occurring infectious diseases? The reason I ask that is because given the threat that is posed by drug-resistant diseases and infections, it seems that those threats should qualify as threats to national security.

MR. AZAR. The threat from drug-resistant bacteria is real. It is important, and we have to be very concerned about the antibiotic pipeline out there. We have to work together with industry to try to make sure that the FDA regulatory process is--this is where the Critical Path Initiative at FDA becomes so important to try to help that pipeline along--streamline for approval to minimize as much as possible, consistent with safety and efficacy, that process. It is where the advanced research and development that we do, and the primary research at NIH, we have focus on this, and then this new effort towards advanced research and development, where we can lend a helping hand on these types of naturally occurring infectious agents. The concern that we have is with Project BioShield itself, $5.6 billion dollars is a lot of money to anyone, but to a pharmaceutical company, and when thinking about developing these types of chemical, biological, radiological/nuclear threat countermeasures, spread around, it doesn't end up being an infinite amount of money. So we have got to prioritize there on the intentional threats. There is a marketplace for antibiotics out there. We need to help encourage it along, and do what we can on primary research and advanced research and development. But unlike the BioShield products, there is a marketplace out there for buying these, if we can just help push them along to help get them developed.

MRS. CUBIN. Right. And do you think that should be part of the BioShield format, if you will?

MR. AZAR. I don't think--

MRS. CUBIN. The pushing along of pharmaceutical companies.

MR. AZAR. The BioShield element itself is limited to simply procuring into the strategic national stockpile. It is about buying products that are ready for licensure. The non-BioShield elements, the primary research at NIH, the advanced research and development that might be out of it, it is not really BioShield itself. I do believe these are areas that, yes, we ought to be focused on naturally occurring areas. For instance, with pandemic, I believe it is $350 million in the 2006 money that Congress appropriated, is precisely going to this type of naturally occurring advanced research and development for agivents that could help do dose structuring on the H5N1 vaccine, and also for that next generation of antiviral drugs, precisely the area you are talking about.

MRS. CUBIN. But if there is not help from the Government, the market is simply not good for antibiotics. Antibiotics, as you know, are drugs that are taken for a very limited amount of time, and the bottom line for a pharmaceutical company simply isn't there to develop new antibiotics. So while I am not saying that necessarily all the money for research should come from NIH, obviously, the pharmaceutical companies have to have a role in that, but I just think that it ought to be identified as a national security problem. Because, in fact, I think the next panel of witnesses will prove, if you will, that it is a national security problem. And I also think that if we find a pathway to being able to deal with these naturally occurring infections and diseases that are getting ahead of us now, that that would be a good blueprint to use for any sort of biological attack that could occur to us, which would fit exactly into your area. Could you describe what types of support HHS provides to smaller firms that do not have adequate funds to follow through in Phase III clinical trials?

MR. AZAR. Well, and that is an excellent question because that is exactly the type of support, that clinical trial support, advanced research and development support that we are asking for $160 million in the 2007, where we could really team with and seed that process along, because it is very expensive, there is often a very high failure rate there for small entities. In particular, it is difficult or impossible for them to absorb all of that cost, and we can share in that risk. I think you have put your finger exactly on the construct of advanced research and development, an area we are getting increasing experience in through pandemic influenza preparedness with the money Congress already has given us and we are implementing, and then the $160 million that we have asked for. This would be the area in the CBRN context for doing precisely that. I think it has been highlighted as a very important issue. Thank you.

MRS. CUBIN. To just go back to the antibiotic situation. What we have been talking about so far is just one incentive for development of new antibiotics, but we need a series of incentives to develop new antibiotics. We need tax credits, patent extensions, FDA-expedited review, plus other things that maybe aren't even on the table yet. And once again, I think that that should be included in HHS's overall plan for the country. I just have one other questions, if you wouldn't mind, Mr. Chairman. What consideration is given to rural areas in formulating countermeasure distribution plans in the event of a bioterror attack? State and local healthcare systems vary from region to region, and in rural areas, in particular, there is a lack of providers. Has any special attention been given to rural care areas?

MR. AZAR. As we have been working with the States on their distribution plans, especially in the pandemic context, we have been focusing the States' energy on developing distribution plans which, of course, for them is statewide. So it is really in their hands on developing those comprehensive plans. What we have been providing through the Cities Readiness Initiative is a separate program to focus some of the extra energies on the complexities of major metropolitan area distribution challenges that we would have, where you have high concentration of individuals. And hopefully, as we learn best practices through that focus and maybe even come up with new better ways of distributing medicines, a tremendous challenge, those will become broadly applicable lessons learned that we can help spread around throughout the country. But I think you are right, we need to keep the focus, but distributing countermeasures is a nationwide issue.

MRS. CUBIN. Thank you and will you keep in mind that cities of population over 50,000, there are only two cities in the entire State of Wyoming, a hundred thousand square miles, so there are special needs out there in rural America. Thank you, Mr. Chairman.

MR. DEAL. Mr. Rogers is recognized for questions.

MR. ROGERS. Thank you, Mr. Chairman. I just want to follow up on Mrs. Cubin's question for a minute. That $160 million you talked about, Mr. Secretary, is that outside of BioShield for advancing drugs, getting them through trials in that?

MR. AZAR. Yes, sir, that is a new money request as part of the 2007 budget, $160 million for advanced research and development. Yes, sir.

MR. ROGERS. And for naturally occurring. So it wouldn't have the same target set, maybe, as a BioShield--

MR. AZAR. No, that $160 million is actually focused on chemical, bio, and radiological/nuclear advanced research and development. It is meant to be in league with the implementation of the BioShield purchasing. It is part of the pulling effort there to get these products closer to the BioShield contracting point.

MR. ROGERS. And just for my own education, how much of the money have you spent that has been allocated for BioShield in 2004?

MR. AZAR. We have obligated, so far, $1.089 billion out of the $5.6 billion Special Reserve Fund. Now, of course, we do have, I believe, four open pending procurements going on right now that would, if they end up in awards, would result in additional obligations of amounts within that.

MR. ROGERS. Okay, so you are asking for $160 million more. You haven't spent all the money since 2004, because I want to make sure I understand that. I won't get into that. My time is short, but I just want to make sure I understand that. You made a statement earlier, and I am confused, because I caught earlier testimony briefly, so please correct me if I am wrong here. But you said that BioShield, when you were answering Mrs. Cubin, was about procurement and stockpiling and buying product that is ready for licensure. If not a direct quote, that is pretty close. Is that correct?

MR. ROGERS. Well, obviously, under BioShield, the products that we acquire, I believe, at the time that we accept them for delivery, they need to be on a track towards final approval by FDA within eight years. So these are products that eventually would need to be on the pathway towards licensure under the BioShield Act.

MR. ROGERS. Okay. Now, is single sourcing of vaccines a good idea?

MR. AZAR. By single sourcing, do you mean--

MR. ROGERS. Sole source, that is it.

MR. AZAR. Sole source contracting?

MR. ROGERS. Yes.

MR. AZAR. Sole source contracting, where there has been no fair and open competition, it would obviously depend on the nature of the market, and that is where we do a request for information to learn about are there even other players in the field. Of the four procurements that we have done under Project BioShield, three of them have been what are called sole source or justification without full and open competition. We have had one procurement, which has been the RPA anthrax vaccine procurement, which was done with full and open competition under the Federal acquisition regulations.

MR. ROGERS. Okay, my question is about, is it good policy to have sole source in vaccines when it comes to bioterrorism? Let me back up. I thought the President was almost visionary when he proposed BioShield. He laid out a niche of a future threat, of which, over time and budget constraints, can get pulled a lot of different ways. And he sat down and said, you know what, this is a real threat that is only going to get worse and we better do it today. And one of the things, as I understand your testimony, is you want to try to expand and we want to take advantage of innovation, and innovation solely happens in sole source contracts. You can't point to too many places in history where sole sourcing of any particular item leads to innovation benefits. As a matter of fact, I would argue that it degrades innovation in that particular area of research. So my understanding of BioShield was to stockpile, which you said that is correct, procurement of something that is likely to be licensured, and according to this $160 million, is to try to find new sources, advancements, and innovation in the field, is that correct?

MR. AZAR. Of course the $160 million is not part of the BioShield. That is--

MR. ROGERS. But you just said a minute ago that it would target some of the vaccines.

MR. AZAR. Oh yes, it is targeting towards bridging the gap between primary research and actual acquisition. I think--

MR. ROGERS. And bridging is a good idea, don't you think?

MR. AZAR. Absolutely.

MR. ROGERS. Good. I want go through just a series of events here that have frustrated me beyond recognition, and I still can't figure out if this is bureaucratic bungling at its best, just lack of interest in what Congress intends, or mismanagement. I can't tell. On April 20 of 2005, myself, Congressman Dingell, Congressman Stupak and Congressman Upton contacted HHS and the Secretary. We expressed concern over the delay of the Department of acquiring a national stockpile for post-exposure and pre-exposure use of FDA licensed anthrax vaccine. Now, they responded back. It took a little longer than we wanted, and said, no, we are going to go ahead and do that, because bridging is important. I think multi-source, bridging, all important stuff, I think, in this. That was April 20 of 2005. On August 4, we contacted the Secretary's office again, Stewart Simonson, regarding a similar purchase of this vaccine, in correlation with the previous letter in conjunction with Mr. Dingell and Mr. Stupak and myself, and they again assured us that this was going to happen. Fall 2005, I had a phone conversation with the Secretary on the progress on the order of those five million additional doses and the commitment was, at that time, he told me it was moving forward and would be done. January 12, 2006, February 15, 2006. March 8, the testimony, the Secretary himself said, let us see, "buy the other five million doses and that we authorized it about a week-and-a-half ago." March 24, I won't get into that.

But as of today, there has been no contracting movement at all, and my argument here is this, and I use this, obviously, because I have probably the most knowledge about this particular area of BioShield, but if this is the way we are operating, it makes complete sense to me that you don't have a strategic plan two years after you have almost $6 billion. That is a fundamental failure to the American people, if you ask me. You are talking about right now setting up a plan, and this is the kind of thing that can exactly happen. Obviously, the concern was enough that you said we need 75 million doses to protect America; good idea. And I am all for new technology. This is recombinant, great. That is fine. That is a wonderful thing. But how many do we have in our stockpile now? Not even close and they have just again asked for an extension. So my argument is it makes no sense to me that you say you are going to do it. You don't do it almost a year later. Either you guys don't know what you are doing--I mean, help me out here. Help me understand why this is such a big issue and a big problem.

MR. AZAR. As you know, the issue here is between two types of anthrax vaccine. There is the old anthrax vaccine absorbed, the AVA vaccine, which we acquired five million doses of and received delivery of it completed in February of 2006, and we have an additional five million option on that. That is the old type of vaccine. And the Institute of Medicine recommended, the interagency scientific body recommended that we move towards the second generation of the RPA, the engineered vaccine, because the hope for greater consistency and greater characterization of the vaccine. As Secretary Leavitt said, exercising the additional five million there, we have stated our intention to exercise that additional five million, subject to the availability of appropriations. As you know, Congress, in Project BioShield, required certain approvals beyond the Secretary of HHS in order to actually implement contracts. We do agree that these procurement procedures need to be faster, more transparent, more effective, and we are working to try to streamline those interagency processes. That is where an upfront strategic plan that is adopted by everybody will allow the implementation of individual procurements to hopefully move much faster through that process. So we share the frustration of the duration that individual procurements take, and we want to work to make that happen more efficiently, Congressman.

MR. ROGERS. With your indulgence, Mr. Chairman, and I understand that. So this is a little bit different answer than we received on April 20, August 4, the fall of 2005, January 12, February: are you all making it up as you go along? I know you can sense my frustration here.

MR. AZAR. And I--

MR. ROGERS. Because I have been told it is fixed, it is done, it is coming, don't worry, about and I wouldn't worry about it. I would take the Secretary, I would take you at your word. I am disappointed that the Secretary didn't show up today. I can understand why. This is an abysmal performance by any standard. I wouldn't expect that I would tell you that I am going to do something that many times, and if I hadn't accomplished it, that you wouldn't be absolutely irate with me. It is not just about me and the issue, it is a fact that we thought that there was a threat big enough in the United States that we are searching for new technology, great, 75 million doses to protect America. That continues to get extended. Okay, we ought be flexible enough to understand that we have to have bridging technology. We should have multiple source in case something like this happens. That was my understanding of BioShield to begin with. And if we are this far behind and this far off and this bureaucratically inept, I am very, very worried about this, and one of the reasons I have called for an investigation. And I was an old FBI agent, and I wasn't the brightest one in the world, but this does not pass the smell test to me.

MR. AZAR. As you know, for anthrax, antibiotics are the front line of defense there and we have dramatically increased the stockpiles. We have enough antibiotics now to treat, post-exposure, I believe it is 780,000 people, and prophalax, with a 60-day course of treatment on antibiotics, 40 million people. That is our frontline defense against an anthrax attack. No vaccine is currently licensed for post-exposure use. They are pre-exposure. So we have five million in the stockpile now for pre-exposure. That would be used for health care workers, other critical personnel, in terms of pre-event vaccination. It is not yet we have an IND, investigational new drug application, at CDC for post-exposure use of the existing vaccine, but it is not an approved product for that and that is part of, in terms of building up this next generation vaccine, part of the requirement there. And the contract, to my understanding, is that it actually be approved for post-exposure vaccination use. And so--

MR. ROGERS. And which I understand the one current supplier, and this really isn't about that, but they in fact have used some therapeutic--the testing, to my understanding, was done through you folks. I guess my whole point is you have made this commitment, which I thought was a good one. You logically said why you want to spend the money for the bridge. It made a lot of sense to me. Why does it take so long? Can you tell me today that this is going to be fixed fairly shortly, or is this number eight and we will be back again soon? If you can help me out on that.

MR. AZAR. I cannot give you a date by which the decision making that is required with the joint secretarial letter of approval, and then the presidential determination of selection will be done.

MR. ROGERS. So when the Secretary authorizes it, and about a week-and-a-half ago, by the way, after they told us that it had already been done, what does that mean?

MR. AZAR. He is one step in the process that the BioShield statute set up that requires several levels of approval on any type of exercise.

MR. ROGERS. And that is between DOD and HHS.

MR. DEAL. The gentleman's time is greatly expired here.

MR. ROGERS. Sure. And, Mr. Chairman, I appreciate your indulgence. I think this is an important issue and I think it shows a huge shortcoming in our effort on BioShield and this ought to scare a lot of us. It certainly scares me. Thank you, Mr. Chairman.

MR. DEAL. Gentlemen, well, thank you for your attendance and your testimony today and we will excuse you at this time. Thank you.

MR. AZAR. Thank you, Mr. Chairman.

MR. DEAL. I will ask Panel two if they will come to the table. Thank you and welcome. Let me introduce the second panel: Dr. Tara O'Toole, CEO and Director of the Center for Biosecurity of the University of Pittsburgh Medical Center; Mr. Peter F. Young, President and CEO of AlphaVax, Incorporated, on behalf of the Biotechnology Industry Organization, Mr. Bruce Cohen, President and CEO of Cellerant Therapeutics, Incorporated, who Ms. Eshoo alluded to earlier, I believe in her statements; Dr. David P. Wright, President and CEO of PharmAthene, and here on behalf of the Alliance for Biosecurity; and Dr. Martin Blaser, President of the Infectious Diseases Society of America. Lady and gentlemen, we are pleased to have you here. Once again, your written testimony is already in the record, and, Dr. O'Toole, I will start with you for your statement.

STATEMENTS OF DR. TARA O'TOOLE, CEO AND DIRECTOR, CENTER FOR BIOSECURITY OF THE UNIVERSITY OF PITTSBURGH MEDICAL CENTER; PETER F. YOUNG, PRESIDENT AND CEO, ALPHAVAX, INC., ON BEHALF OF BIOTECHNOLOGY INDUSTRY ORGANIZATION; BRUCE COHEN, PRESIDENT AND CEO, CELLERANT THERAPEUTICS, INC.; DR. DAVID P. WRIGHT, PRESIDENT AND CEO, PHARMATHENE, ON BEHALF OF

ALLIANCE FOR BIOSECURITY; AND DR. MARTIN BLASER, PRESIDENT, INFECTIOUS DISEASES SOCIETY OF AMERICA.

DR. O'TOOLE. I appreciate the opportunity to speak on this important topic. I represent the Center for Biosecurity at the University of Pittsburgh Medical Center. We have been working since 1998 on the issues of biodefense, which I know all the members of this committee agree are of critical importance to national security. The prior discussion, I think, was very interesting and illustrated both the essential importance of the BioShield legislation that was passed a few years ago, as well as the complexity of this issue. At the core of the questions about what do we buy, when, and how much do we buy, and what should we invest in technologies versus which of the existing countermeasures should be put in the stockpile, is a question of cost. It is my view that we are still, as a country, thinking about biodefense on the wrong scale. We are thinking about it as another health problem as opposed to a major national security threat.

BioShield was an important piece of legislation. It is a very good start, but it is not nearly enough money for the purpose that has to be served. We are off by about a magnitude of order right now. And that cost is going to go up as the threat of bio-weapons emerges more clearly, and that will include the emergence of bioengineered weapons, which are probably viable today. We need to recognize that the problem biopharma is having engaging in this process is partly about opportunity costs. They simply make lots more money, not just two or three times more money, but ten or a hundred times more money investing in stuff that does not have to do with infectious disease. This is true whether you are talking about drugs against biological weapons-induced diseases or drugs against naturally occurring infections. And what we are seeing is the biopharma industry, as a whole, fleeing from investments in anti-infectives, in vaccines, antibiotics, and so forth. We need to do something about this. This is a strategic problem. I think the most important part of it for national security's sake is no doubt bioterrorism. But as the congresswoman noted, the rise of antibiotic-resistant bugs and so forth is also a real issue, and we are going to have to figure out a way to spend more money in the future on this critical problem.

Now, I think HHS has done work in trying to step up and implement this new legislation, but the fact of the matter is, biodefense generally and the procurement of new drugs and vaccines and the investment in whole new areas of drugs and vaccines is a new mission for HHS. They have lots of good people working their hearts out over there trying to administer BioShield, but they fall far short of what is needed. We need more people at HHS, a lot more, I would say a hundred more just to administer BioShield appropriately, and they need to have the right expertise. We need people at HHS who have experience in the biopharma field and who have managed complex, long-term acquisition contracts, such as DOD does all the time, but HHS has never done heretofore.

And finally, I think we are going to rapidly run out of the strategy of trying to find a drug or a vaccine against each bug that might present a biological weapons threat. We are going to be faced in the future with unanticipated threats, some of the bioengineered agents that come upon us and to which we have to respond very quickly. Right now, it takes about ten years to create a new drug. We need, as a matter of national security strategy, to start instituting research projects in partnership with the biopharma industry that can radically reduce how long it takes to develop a drug. We need to go from ten years to about two weeks. We can do this if we apply our know how across the spectrum of drug development, from improving R and D to helping us through this middle phase valley of death to improving clinical trial efficiencies to getting our regulatory apparatus even more efficient than it is now. We need to take this project on as a matter of high national security priority and we can do it, but that is going to take some time. In the meanwhile, we have to stockpile drugs, but this notion of having a cupboard full of drugs for all of the possible biological weapons agents, especially for the bioengineered agents that are upon us, is not going to be viable, even for the United States of America for very much longer. It is a stopgap measure that we need to take, but we need to take the next step into this new strategic world of radically accelerating drug development. Thank you, Mr. Chairman.

[The prepared statement of Dr. Tara O'Toole follows:]

PREPARED STATEMENT OF DR. TARA O'TOOLE, CEO AND DIRECTOR, CENTER FOR BIOSECURITY OF THE UNIVERSITY OF PITTSBURGH MEDICAL CENTER

Mr. Chairman, Congressman Dingell, and members of the committee, thank you for the opportunity to address the vital issue of biodefense and the difficult challenges surrounding the US government's efforts to procure medicines and vaccines against biological agents that could be used in terrorist attacks against US civilians. My name is Tara O'Toole. I am the Director and CEO of the Center for Biosecurity of the University of Pittsburgh Medical Center and a professor of medicine at the University of Pittsburgh Medical School. The Center for Biosecurity is a non-profit, non-partisan, multidisciplinary organization located in Baltimore which includes physicians, public health professionals, and biological and social scientists. The Center is dedicated to understanding the threat of large-scale, lethal epidemics due to bioterrorism and natural causes. My colleagues and I are committed to the development of policies and practices that would help prevent bioterrorist attacks or destabilizing natural epidemics, and, should prevention fail, would mitigate the destructive consequences of such events.

For several years now, the Center for Biosecurity has been working in collaboration with academia, industry, and government to stimulate development and procurement of new medicines and vaccine for biodefense. In March 2005, we initiated the formation of the Alliance for Biosecurity, a collaboration between the Center and leading biotechnology and pharmaceutical companies with the intention of working together in the public interest to promote the creation of a robust and sustainable biomedical research and development infrastructure that we believe is needed to prevent and treat the infectious disease threats that present US and global security challenges in the 21st century. These threats include large-scale epidemics of natural disease as well as bioterrorist attacks using conventional or bioengineered weapons.

Biological weapons have been proven to work, are capable of causing massive lethality, are relatively cheap, and are increasingly easy to design, build and disseminate. We are in the midst of a bioscientific revolution that will make building and using biological weapons even more deadly and increasingly easy. Finally, the materials and technical know-how needed to make a bioweapon that could infect hundreds of thousands of people are already widely distributed around the planet, and the number of people who possess the expertise needed to create bioweapons is rapidly growing as biotechnology and pharmaceutical research and production expand into developing countries.

Preventing either a natural epidemic or a bioterrorist attack is, unfortunately, unlikely. Therefore, the nation's ability to rapidly and effectively respond in the face of a biosecurity crisis should be a central pillar in our biosecurity strategy. The nation's response to an outbreak must be designed to prevent potentially destabilizing social, economic, and political consequences, in addition to preventing illness and death on a large scale. Medicines and vaccines that can counter illnesses caused by exposure to bioweapons agents are obviously an essential component of biodefense and would be critical to controlling the spread of contagious disease. A recent report from the Institute of Medicine found that the array of biological agents that pose a significant threat to biosecurity is much larger and more diverse than any of today's "threat lists."[1] Yet, since 2001, the US has acquired only a single countermeasure – smallpox vaccine. Why is this?

Funding for biodefense countermeasures is not comprehensive and is not commensurate with the threat of bioattacks.

Thus far, the US government has focused efforts to acquire biodefense countermeasures on basic research investments and on Bioshield funding for acquisition of countermeasures that are sufficiently advanced that they are eligible for Investigative New Drug (IND) status. What's missing from the US government's biodefense funding strategy is support during the so-called "valley of death", the crucial middle phase of drug development between basic research and acquisition of final products (see figure).

[1] "Globalization, Biosecurity, and the Future of the Life Sciences," Institute of Medicine, January 2006.

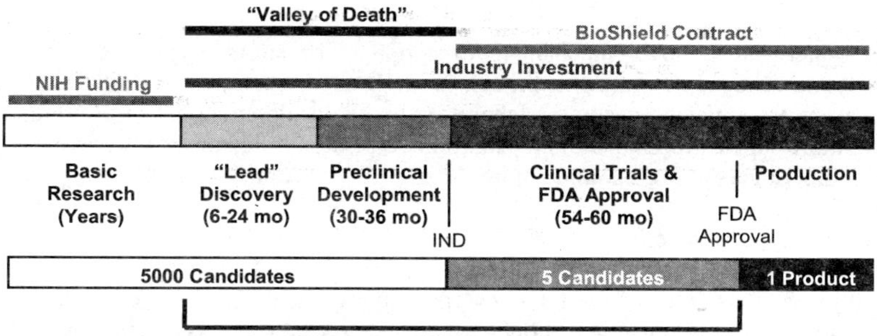

Lead Discovery to FDA Approval: 8-12 Years
(This timeline is for development of medicines/drugs, length of vaccine development is similar.)

Drug and vaccine development is an expensive, high risk undertaking. Of 5000 drug "candidates" identified by scientists, only 5 make it to clinical trials and only one of these, on average, will become a licensed product.[2] The lack of support from the US government during the crucial intermediate stages of development results in premature failures of potential countermeasures as biopharma companies struggle to maintain operations through long periods of uncertainty without outside support. The priorities of the private capital markets, instead of the priorities of government, are driving products through the "valley of death." Unfortunately, countermeasure development is unattractive to private investors because there are no markets outside of governments for most of these products, and even in the most profitable scenarios, biodefense countermeasures – as with anti-infectives generally – cannot generate profits comparable to successful medicines for chronic disease that are taken for years by large populations.[3] This is one of the prime reasons that there are only 5 major vaccine manufacturers left in the world. One expert in drug development was quoted in a 2004 study performed by the Center for Biosecurity and the Sarnoff Corporation as saying:

> *"You make a new antibiotic and if it's really terrific you'll have peak sales of $300–500 million per year. If you make a drug for cancer that extends life by 4 months, you can charge $40,000 per dose. The difference is so staggering...."*[4]

Without some form of government support for the "valley of death," perhaps in the form of grants, contracts, or significant milestone payments such as the Department of Defense uses in the acquisition of complex weapons systems, few companies will be able to secure outside financing or invest their own capital in countermeasure development.

Government-funded basic research is an essential part of biodefense strategy, partly because research into infectious diseases has, in recent times, been less well funded by the private-sector than research for cancer and other types of illness (HIV/AIDS is the exception). As noted, the private sector has been systematically abandoning R&D investments in infectious disease generally because other investment opportunities are much more lucrative.[5] As a result of industry's retreat from infectious disease research, there is less innovation. Since 1998, FDA has approved just 10 new antibiotics – only

---

[2] "2004 Survey: Medicines in Development for Infectious Diseases," PhRMA, 2004; Nwaka, S. and R.G. Ridley "Virtual drug discovery and development for neglected infectious diseases through public-private partnerships," *Nature Reviews Drug Discovery*, vol. 2, p. 919-28, 2003.

[3] "Bad Bugs, No Drugs," Report from the Infectious Diseases Society of America, July 2004; Kennedy, D., "Drug Discovery" (editorial), *Science*, vol. 303, p. 1729, 2004.

[4] Gilfillan, L. *et al.*, "Taking the Measure of Countermeasures: Leaders' Views on the Nation's Capacity to Develop Biodefense Countermeasures," *Biosecurity and Bioterrorism*, vol. 2, p. 320-27, 2004.

[5] "Bad Bugs, No Drugs," Report from the Infectious Diseases Society of America, July 2004.

two of which had a novel mechanism of action.[6] The strong support Congress has accorded basic biodefense research though the NIH should continue. Efforts to facilitate the transition from discoveries in the laboratory to the development of useful products by offering more support to innovators trying to traverse the "valley of death" could result in many more success stories and more "bang for the buck" from basic research investments.

With the passage of the 2004 Bioshield legislation (P.L. 108-276), the nation undertook to pay for the acquisition of countermeasures. The Bioshield Purchase Fund of $5.6 billion sounds like a lot of money, particularly in the context of public health expenditures. But it is not much money when viewed as a necessary national security investment. A single Nimitz class aircraft carrier costs about $4 billion; ten such ships have been built for the US Navy. The size of the Bioshield procurement fund must also be examined in light of the actual costs of drug development: it is estimated that the average out-of-pocket cost of developing a new drug is $400 million; if opportunity costs are included, the cost is $800 million.[7] A more recent study calculates the costs of drug development could be even higher.[8] Indeed, the first Bioshield contract, for 75 million doses of recombinant anthrax vaccine, amounted to $877 million. The reality is that $5.6 billion will not go far, particularly when the entire threat spectrum is considered and the costs of actually acquiring (not just developing) medicines and vaccines are contemplated.

Current HHS Structure and Staffing Levels Need to be Strengthened

Biodefense is a relatively new and complex mission for the Department of Health and Human Services (HHS). Although many competent people within HHS are working hard to manage countermeasure development and acquisition, too few federal staff, many with little relevant experience, are trying to do too much under ferocious time pressures. It is imperative that HHS be granted the authority to hire about 100 new staff, many of them at the senior level, to manage these important programs. It is especially important that HHS hire people with experience in drug and vaccine development and production.

The current processes associated with threat identification, countermeasure development and acquisition are poorly coordinated, slow moving, confusing and often contrary to routine business practices. This is due in part to the number of different agencies involved (OPHEP, ORD, FDA, NIH, DHS). But it is also the case that HHS lacks experience managing complicated, long-term acquisition projects such as DOD handles routinely. The Federal government has chosen to pursue biodefense countermeasures through partnerships with the biopharma industry. Such an approach is a sensible way to make efficient use of the prodigious know-how and resources of the private sector. But for this approach to work, the Federal government must be a reliable partner. From biopharma's perspective – and the perspective of investors – it is critical that the government maintain a transparent, predictable process with clear timelines, explicit liability protection and fair compensation rights, and develop predictable rules for the protection of intellectual property rights. Failure to recognize these realities means that few companies will choose to pursue countermeasure development and production, and the country will not have the medicines it needs in times of crisis.

After the terrorist attacks of 2001, HHS was tasked to take on a welter of new missions related to homeland security. The management structure and staffing of HHS

---

[6] Spellberg, B. *et al.*, "Trends in antimicrobial drug development: implications for the future," *Clinical Infectious Diseases*, vol. 38, p 1279–86, 2004.

[7] DiMasi, J.A. *et al.*, "The price of innovation: new estimates of drug development costs," *Journal of Health Economics*, vol. 22, p151–185, 2003.

[8] Adams, C.P and V.V. Brantner, "Estimating The Cost Of New Drug Development: Is It Really $802 Million?", *Health Affairs*, vol. 25, p. 420-28, 2006.

has simply not kept pace with these assignments. HHS is larger in dollar terms than the Department of Defense – and yet HHS does not have a single undersecretary. Secretary Leavitt has noted that he has 27 direct reports – a situation he recognizes as "not at all an ideal organizational structure."

Cabinet Secretaries should have broad discretion in how their agencies are organized, but I believe that Congress should consider authorizing HHS to establish at least one – or better, two or three – Undersecretary positions. This would provide the agency with more senior managers capable of coordinating HHS's vast programmatic span of control. In the realm of public health preparedness, an Undersecretary for Public Health (which could be combined with the present Assistant Secretary for Health or the position of Surgeon General) could better coordinate the varying HHS programs now spread among the Assistant Secretary for OPHEP, CDC, HRSA, NIH, AHRQ, and ONCHIT. In addition, an Undersecretary would be better able to represent HHS in the interagency process.

Focus on Accelerated Development of Countermeasures

The US does not yet have a coherent biodefense strategy, nor do we have a strategy for countermeasure research, development, and production that takes account of the full spectrum of possible bioweapons agents, including engineered threats. It is clear that a handful of pathogens such as anthrax, smallpox, plague, etc. are at the top of most threat lists because of their availability, lethality, contagiousness, historic development as bioweapons, etc. Developing and stockpiling specific countermeasures against these high-priority threats is a rational and pressing national security need.

However, in the long term, the current approach of developing countermeasures against each potential bioweapon agent will prove futile. Natural outbreaks of novel infectious diseases (e.g. SARS) are commonplace, and there are dozens of naturally occurring pathogens which could serve as bioweapons agents today. Moreover, the ongoing revolution in bioscience will enable the creation of more and more bioweapons agents covering an enlarging spectrum of targets.[9] As the "threat space" expands, it will become increasingly difficult and costly to use a "one-bug-one-drug" strategy to define the appropriate armamentarium of countermeasures that must be developed and stockpiled – and perhaps never used. In addition, the country will have to confront the specter of covert bioattacks using heretofore unanticipated bioengineered agents. Avoiding the destabilizing effects of a large-scale, lethal campaign of such attacks will require the ability to rapidly design, develop and produce new countermeasures from a standing start – in weeks, if not days. The need to anticipate and prepare for such bioengineered weapons is not in the far-off future. We are already living in the age of bioengineering. Scientists estimate that in five years it will be possible to synthesize any virus from non-living components.

A major strategic goal of US biosecurity strategy should be the radical acceleration of drug and vaccine development. The US government should embark on an ambitious program to incrementally reduce drug development and production time across the entire development spectrum. Important reductions in development time might be achieved across the timeline of drug and vaccine development with efforts such as:

- technology improvements such as in silico modeling, genomics, and synthetic biology;
- wider sharing of, and access to, improved research tools such as toxicological databases, test-tube and animal models of diseases, chemical libraries of possible medicines, and high throughput screening of potential drug candidates;

---

[9] Petro, J.B., T.R. Plasse, J.A. McNulty, "Biotechnology: Impact on Biological Warfare and Biodefense," *Biosecurity and Bioterrorism*, vol. 1, p. 161-68, 2003.

- more efficient clinical testing, such as might be accomplished with integrated electronic health records;
- streamlined regulatory review such as might be achieved by adding staff and leadership in FDA and developing policies that account for the unique aspects of biodefense countermeasures;
- the creation of public-private consortia to facilitate sharing of information between developers, to address predictive safety testing (i.e. to focus on scientific ways to predict toxicity), and to tackle other key countermeasure development challenges.

This is not just about developing new technologies. The US government will need to foster new systems to enable private sector developers – many of whom are direct competitors – to work together with the government and academia so that we can take advantage of the complete storehouse of knowledge and expertise available.

If the US were to undertake an ambitious long-term effort to focus on accelerated countermeasures development, it is likely to be successful. The US currently has the advantage in bioscience expertise and experience – invaluable assets that could be well leveraged in such an effort, although we are also rapidly outsourcing most drug and vaccine development overseas, mostly to India and China.

Success in such a venture would bring many benefits in addition to forming the foundation of a coherent and sustainable biodefense strategy. In biopharma, time is money; the average drug now requires a decade to develop from concept to licensed product. Learning how to accelerate countermeasure development would necessarily mean that the costs of countermeasures would decrease, probably substantially. This effect would have direct implications for the costs of pharmaceuticals generally – even during "peacetime" – thereby reducing health care costs and placing the cost of vital drugs and vaccines within reach of developing countries.

Such a program of accelerated drug development should proceed in partnership with biopharma companies in the private sector, much as the Department of Defense developed partnerships with major military contractors. If such a project was ambitious enough, and properly structured and financed, and if the Federal government made a long-term commitment to such a project, it is likely that the leaders of biopharma would agree to participate.

It would not be easy to achieve radical acceleration of countermeasure production. But incremental progress is almost certain, and would over time have potentially significant impacts. I am convinced that such a project will be undertaken; the remaining question is whether the US will make such a commitment before we experience a large-scale bioevent, such as a terrorist attack or a naturally occurring pandemic, or after.

The Biodefense and Pandemic Vaccine and Drug Development Act (S. 1873) being proposed by Senator Burr as a next step beyond Bioshield is not perfect. It is a modest bill that will not transform countermeasure R&D or dramatically reshape HHS. But it is an extremely useful piece of legislation and should be enacted into law. The bill makes important incremental improvements in the structure of HHS, allowing the agency to acquire competent staff and bring more clarity and transparency to its countermeasure procurement processes. It provides mechanisms for supporting companies in the "valley of death", in a manner similar to the DOD acquisition process and appropriate to the development of complex products with limited markets. The related bill being proposed by Senator Kennedy (S. 1880) also makes the point that improvements in the current approach to countermeasure development are needed. These bills send the message that the US government is concerned about biodefense and wants to improve countermeasure development. Should the Congress fail to pass meaningful Bioshield legislation this session, there is a real danger that the biopharma industry will read this as a clear message: Congress is not serious about biodefense.

MR. DEAL. Thank you. Mr. Young?

MR. YOUNG. Mr. Chairman, thank you for the opportunity to testify before the committee today. AlphaVax is a small 70-person, privately held R and D stage biotechnology company based in North Carolina, and we are working to develop and commercialize a vaccine technology, a platform technology, and I am here today testifying on behalf of BIO.

Since 2002, AlphaVax has received four NIH peer-reviewed biodefense vaccine early-development grants. These grants represent about $38 million in total awards, and it is our long-term goal to use these grants, BioShield monies, and if commercially viable, private capital to develop bioterrorism countermeasures. If it weren't for Project BioShield and the Government's grant funding in this arena, my company would not be working on biodefense vaccine targets at all. We have no sales. We have no profit. The only money we have is money from people who believe we might be able to produce important new vaccines one day. That is a long, costly, and inherently uncertain process. We have limited amounts of time, people, and money with which to deliver on these expectations.

As we consider the pressing need to improve preparedness, we must recognize the enormous challenges intrinsic in that and the successes to date. The public/private sector partnership necessary to protect the Nation from bioterrorism and pandemic threats is unprecedented in the area of biopharmaceutical development, and it must have an entrepreneurial and innovative spirit. Dedicated personnel, and we have heard today from many agencies who have already devoted countless hours to build the effort from the ground up, and these efforts and accomplishments ought to be recognized, and HHS has given examples of contracts that are already underway. However, as important as these contributions are, more must be done. Essential reforms to the BioShield partnership are necessary to better enable the successful development of biodefense and pandemic countermeasures. Incremental change can increase capacity for existing products or achieve modest improvements on existing countermeasures, but to achieve dramatic success BioShield needs to adopt a culture and methodology consistent with innovation, the innovation it wants to stimulate. This is an approach that is modeled in the private sector by a technology investment.

I am going to emphasize just three areas. First, Congress must reform Project BioShield to fill the important funding gap that has been alluded to between early development and the ultimate commercial marketing of a product, which companies like mine without self-funded R and D refer to as the valley of death, with good reason. The development process for drugs and biologics is complex, time consuming, costly, and high risk. There are added challenges to that in developing countermeasures, and these countermeasure opportunities compete for investment dollars with other markets. The Government is usually the only purchaser for countermeasures and because of all of this, it is extremely difficult for small companies to raise private funding to cover the costs incurred after early stage NIH funding but before the Government begins paying for a final product. So to address the funding gap, BioShield ought to reform to allow the sharing of risk between industry and the Government during the entire course of product development, and funding to bridge that advanced development valley of death is a key element to a successful and meaningful partnership.

A second recommendation would improve the coordination and also the character of the staffing that animates the Government activity in this. The partnership required for successful countermeasure development includes a number of different agencies, and each plays a role in the process. The objectives and requirements of the various agencies must obviously be aligned and coordinated with contract solicitation terms and be part of an early dialogue. The expectations of regulators for licensure and emergency use authorization ought to be coordinated with the contract terms. Ambiguous, additional, and unforeseen requirements that arise outside of contract terms magnify companies' financial risk. Clear and strong leadership, with a fundamental understanding of biotechnology development, is required to coordinate the many agencies and objectives and to ensure that development is not choked by bureaucracy or inexperience. The challenges and complex nature of countermeasure development, coupled with the urgent need to prepare, require that critical staff level positions be adequately funded. HHS needs not only sufficient resources to expedite the procurement processes, but flexible hiring authorities are needed to staff key positions with the expertise and understanding of the pharmaceutical industry, both small and large companies that animate it.

The final point of emphasis is just the need to clearly and predictably identify future needs. Countermeasures can't be developed in the absence of clear and reliable articulation of the needs and commitments. Effective product development requires an understanding of the end goal, and to date there have been too few material threat assessments that have resulted in requests for proposals and acquisitions. There have also been instances where expected needs were dramatically reduced upon solicitation of the contract. Lack of clarity and predictability of technical requirements can further frustrate planning and execution. To enable an effective public/private partnership, requirements ought to be developed through dialogue with industry and there must be a shared understanding of objectives, purchase solicitations, and the consideration of the complexities of the industry and the development process.

In conclusion, BioShield has been an important first step. Enactment of some of the more modest reforms I have alluded to will spur more bioterrorism and pandemic countermeasure participation by the private sector, but without reform and additional funding, that participation will still fall short. Many companies like mine will have no choice but to avoid the biodefense valley of death and many promising countermeasures will never progress. Our industry is based on a productive relationship and understanding of the link between risk and innovation, and to achieve similar productivity and countermeasures, BioShield needs an approach that cultivates innovation. Thank you.

[The prepared statement of Peter F. Young follows:]

PREPARED STATEMENT OF PETER F. YOUNG, PRESIDENT AND CEO, ALPHAVAX, INC., ON BEHALF OF BIOTECHNOLOGY INDUSTRY ORGANIZATION

Good afternoon and thank you for the opportunity to testify before the Committee today on behalf of BIO, the Biotechnology Industry Organization. My name is Peter Young, and I am the President & Chief Executive of AlphaVax, Inc. AlphaVax is a privately held pre-revenue biotechnology company based in North Carolina that is working to develop and commercialize a vaccine technology that was originally invented in part at the US Army Medical Research Institute for Infectious Diseases. In addition to vaccine development funding we receive from the Division of AIDS in the National Institute of Allergy and Infectious Diseases (NIAID) at the National Institutes of Health (NIH), my company has since 2002 received four NIH peer-reviewed biodefense vaccine early development grants for the Marburg virus, botulinum toxin, viral encephalitis viruses, and small pox, as well as grants against SARS and pandemic influenza. These six grants represent $38 million in total awards, not including clinical support funded separately by the NIH on some of the programs. My company consists of 70 people.

BIO represents more than 1,100 biotechnology companies, academic institutions, state biotechnology centers and related organizations across the United States and 31 other nations. BIO members are involved in the research and development of healthcare, agricultural, industrial and environmental biotechnology products

I wish to preface my general remarks by noting that if it were not for Project Bioshield and the government's grant funding in this arena, my company would not be working on biodefense vaccine targets at all. We have no sales and no profit: the only money we have is money from people who believe we might be able to produce important new vaccines for diseases they are interested in. Biotechnology companies like mine have a limited amount of time, people, and money with which to show they can deliver on these expectations. If they don't deliver, they can't attract investment capital, and they die. If I were a big company with my own sales and profits, I would have a little more leeway, but I would still be critically answerable to the expectations of investors and the capital markets.

The intrinsic risks and costs of developing biodefense vaccines are not different from other vaccines the private sector invests in. However, to justify working on biodefense vaccines, the private sector – big company or small - must ask itself additional questions before pursuing countermeasures:

- Is the potential market big enough to be attractive?
- Are the risks no greater?
- Are the costs subsidized or covered?
- Are there technical or financial leverages that advance the technology?

If the answer to these questions are negative or absent compared to other opportunities, companies won't participate.

As we consider the progress to date in medical countermeasure development and the actions needed to improve preparedness, we must recognize the enormous challenges and the successes to date. The magnitude of the public-private partnership necessary to protect the nation from bioterrorist and pandemic threats is unprecedented in the area of biopharmaceutical development. This is an enormous task for the Department of Homeland Security (DHS) and the Department of Health and Human Services (HHS) and its agencies, and much hard work by dedicated individuals was needed to build the initiative from the ground up several years ago. These efforts and accomplishments must be recognized. HHS has contracts underway for vaccines for anthrax and countermeasures for acute radiation syndrome and other radiological indications. Over 180 million doses of a smallpox vaccine have been delivered to the Strategic National Stockpile. Additionally, NIH, through NIAID, has issued numerous grants for millions of dollars that have been essential to spur early stage research in biodefense products. Grants have also been issued to foster the construction of biosafety containment facilities necessary for the research and development of countermeasures for harmful pathogens. Dedicated personnel from many agencies have devoted countless hours to this effort in national security.

However, as important as these contributions have been, more must be done. Essential enhancements to the commitment of a public-private partnership are necessary to enable the successful development of biodefense and pandemic countermeasures. The urgency of timing must be reinforced. As a nation we have faced a heightened threat of terrorist attacks, and the threat of an influenza pandemic and news of the spread of avian influenza grows each day. We must approach these reforms with a recognition that we currently do not have nearly enough vaccine and therapeutics to protect all Americans from a pandemic. With this in mind, I would like to offer perspectives on three key areas of need:

- Clear and predictable identification of needs that are developed in a public/private partnership with dialogue.
- Strong leadership and coordination.
- Strong and predictable funding that addresses both development and acquisition of critical medical countermeasures.

In order to understand what changes are necessary to better engage industry in the development of medical countermeasures, an understanding of the factors that affect the drug development process is helpful. The development process for drugs and biologics is complex, time-consuming, and costly. It often involves many partners through different stages, and it includes a number of complicated intellectual property and licensing agreements. The development of a biopharmaceutical product can cost tens or hundreds of millions of dollars and take years from initial research to commercialization.

Companies interested in drug development typically engage in sophisticated market analysis to assess what demands exist for products before engaging in costly and time-consuming research and development. An understanding of the market is important not just at the time of manufacturing and sale - it is a critical component that drives risk assessments through the product development cycle. Because the costs of drug development generally increase substantially as the product moves from one phase to the next, careful risk assessments are made during all phases of development. It is a reality that the stability and robustness of the final market is a key determinant in these risk assessments and the viability of product development.

Understanding of the final market includes information on volume of demand and economic factors. But important technical considerations are also incorporated into the development cycle. For example, the mode of administration, dose and formulation requirements, and shelf-life requirements are important factors in product development.

Uncertainty in these specifications, or a change late in the development cycle, can have a profound impact on risk assessments, and ultimately the time and cost of development. It is also important to recognize that even with clear market needs, few products move from early development to licensure without some technical changes. This is expected, as a goal of advanced development is to optimize the product for the best effectiveness and safety.

While these considerations exist for all biopharmaceutical development, biodefense and pandemic products face heightened challenges. The government will generally be the only or primary purchaser, and thus will set the market demands. Lack of clarity and stability of government requirements translates directly to lack of clarity and stability in development goals. This in turn has a direct impact on whether or not companies can step forward and contribute the expertise of the private sector.

Biodefense and pandemic products also face increased risks for liability claims, so liability protections and an injury compensation program are necessary to spur industry to participate in these challenging markets at the government's request. These products will likely be administered in the face of an emergency to otherwise healthy individuals. Companies must be assured that they will not face financial ruin due to unforeseen and unavoidable adverse reactions. The Public Readiness and Emergency Preparations Act (PREP Act), passed as part of the 2006 Defense Appropriations Act, provides responsible liability protections, coupled with a compensation program for those injured by medical countermeasures. It is important to note that liability protections are necessary to enable all stages of development – not just final sale of product. Small companies must attract investors and capital to move products through the development cycle. The ability to attract such capital is severely constrained if strong, responsible, and stable liability protections are not in place.

Bearing in mind these factors that influence biopharmaceutical investment decisions and the competition for investment dollars, there are a number of critical and inter-dependent areas that need to be addressed. Incentives must be in place to both engage and sustain industry participation in this important partnership.

<u>First, we need clear and predictable identification of needs that are developed in a public/private partnership with dialogue and coordination</u>. A predictable demand is needed to allow companies to consider and assess their ability to enter this market. Without this, the ambiguity and uncertainty will cause investment dollars to be directed to other efforts. As noted earlier, effective product development requires an understanding of the end goal.

To date, there have been only a handful of material threat assessments that have resulted in requests for proposals (RFPs) and acquisitions. There have also been instances where expected needs were dramatically reduced upon solicitation of a contract. Lack of clarity and predictability of technical requirements, such as expiry dating and filling and storage requirements, can further frustrate planning and execution. This creates uncertainty in the market, and severely challenges business planning necessary for commercialization of countermeasures. Demand drives the product development process, and realistic requirements, developed with dialogue with industry, need to be incorporated early into the drug development process. Countermeasures cannot be developed in the absence of clear and reliable articulation of needs and commitments to purchase successfully developed products.

To enable an effective public/private partnership, requirements should be developed through dialogue with industry. It is essential that industry and government have a shared understanding of objectives, and that purchase solicitations are developed in a framework that addresses the complexities of the biopharmaceutical industry and contain the appropriate level of specifications and delivery terms.

<u>Second, strong leadership, coordination, and sufficient funding and flexibility in staffing are essential to success</u>. The public/private partnership required for successful

countermeasure development includes numerous government departments and agencies, each playing a key role in the process. The objectives and requirements of the various agencies must be aligned and coordinated with solicitation terms and must be part of the early dialogue. These activities include funding for early and late stage research and development, regulatory support, and contract management. For example, production and delivery of products are inherently affected by regulatory requirements. The expectations of regulators for licensure and emergency use authorization should be coordinated with the contract terms. Ambiguous, additional and unforeseen requirements that arise outside of contract terms magnify companies' financial risk. Strong and clear leadership is required to coordinate the many agencies and objectives.

Also, the challenges and complex nature of countermeasure development, coupled with the urgent need to prepare, require that critical staff level positions be adequately funded and staffed. In order to sufficiently expedite the procurement processes, HHS needs sufficient resources. Flexible hiring authorities can also help ensure that key positions are staffed with expertise and understanding of the biopharmaceutical industry and the functioning of both small and large companies. In order for a true public/private partnership to succeed, both sides must be resourced to rapidly address the full array of development issues with experienced judgment to reach effective, expeditious outcomes.

Third, the funding for biodefense and pandemic countermeasures must be strong and consistent, and should recognize the shared-risk of a public/private partnership. A comprehensive preparedness strategy is needed that addresses the various threats for which we must prepare, and sufficient funding to achieve their commercialization. Potentially life-saving products are at risk of dying in the gap between the "push" of early stage development and "pull" of commercialization – a gap referred to as the "Valley of Death".

Shared risk in advanced development should be incorporated into the funding plans, as it is another important element of a successful public/private partnership, and critical to bridging the "Valley of Death". Biopharmaceutical development is inherently risky, and as noted earlier, costs go up significantly through each development phase. Because of this, companies carefully evaluate investment decisions at each phase. Important products for biodefense and pandemic preparedness may not survive these risk calculations without sufficient government partnering and transparency in interactions with government entities.

In non-biodefense/non-pandemic markets, in which there is a "natural" market for products without government participation, venture capitalists, partnering companies, and company equity are vehicles used to fuel the development of these expensive phases based on marketing and risk-assessment forecasts. It is very difficult to attract and justify these vehicles for biodefense and pandemic products in the absence of a predictable and robust market. Even with clear and predictable identification of government needs, the reality is that the overall market for many of these life-saving products that are essential to national security may be relatively small.

Because of this, many promising technologies stall in early and mid-stage development, not due to technical failure, but because the market "pull" is not sufficient. Again, it is important to recall that biodefense and pandemic countermeasures must compete for investment dollars that can be directed to other markets. Funding of advanced development to bridge the "Valley of Death" is a key element in a successful and meaningful effort to produce countermeasures essential for our national security.

The comprehensive strategy should include an appropriate array of diagnostics, preventatives, and therapies against threat agents. Research tools that facilitate our understanding of targeted pathogens and facilitate product development are also an important component of a comprehensive strategy.

The task before us is large. Prior to the events of 9/11 and the subsequent anthrax attacks that fall, there was no significant demand for biodefense products for the civilian population. Facing the growing threat of an influenza pandemic, based on our current vaccine technology and manufacturing capabilities, we are currently simply unable to produce enough vaccine for all Americans. The good news is that with sufficient investment, promising biotechnologies in development offer potential advances in multiple dimensions. New recombinant and cell-culture vaccine technologies have the potential to greatly enhance capacity and production efficiencies. New antivirals are being developed with the potential to treat multiple strains of influenza, and diagnostic tools are in development to rapidly detect bioterrorist agents and pandemic strains and allow for faster response and containment efforts.

When considering the cost of funding countermeasure development and purchase, full consideration must be given to the cost of not making this investment – in terms of lives, health, and economic costs. For example, economists from the CDC have estimated that the impact of a pandemic in the United States could be 90,000 to 200,000 deaths, hundreds of thousands of hospitalizations, and tens of millions of outpatient visits and illnesses. They estimate the economic impact in our country could be between $71 billion to $166 billion – excluding disruptions to commerce and society.[1] A World Bank leading economist estimated that the worldwide cost of an influenza pandemic could be $800 billion, with $550 billion of this affecting industrialized nations.[2] The costs to life, health, and the economy could be overwhelming, and these staggering numbers don't express the societal challenge of recovery.

Additionally, the public health synergies of investing in robust anti-infective and diagnostic markets must be recognized. If a pandemic does not arise or a bioterrorist event does not occur by a certain date, our investments should not be considered misguided. These investments should be viewed as a pathway to securing our future and assuring that the United States will be poised to deal with future threats. In addition to responsibly preparing for public health emergencies and national security, new technologies and manufacturing and infrastructure capacities fostered through these efforts will likely yield public health benefits in other infectious diseases that face market challenges.

Investments are also needed in animal models and other research tools. Pandemic and biodefense countermeasure development is characterized by constraints on human efficacy trials, tight controls of pathogen agents, and rapid changes in potentially pandemic strains. Because of this, the development of knowledge and tools that will allow us to anticipate, approximate, and characterize the agents, and model the effects of the agents and their countermeasures in humans, is an essential part of pandemic and biodefense preparedness. In addition to animal models, investments in assay development and standardization, correlates of protection, predictive toxicology, host response, and other tools are an important part of an effective countermeasures program. As with the countermeasures themselves, the market for research and diagnostic tools in this area has generally been too uncertain and too small to warrant any significant investment by commercial firms.

In conclusion, enactment of the modest reforms outlined above will spur bioterrorism and pandemic countermeasure development more than is the case at this moment. Because of Project BioShield, more companies like mine are now doing research into these countermeasures. Without reform, however, clarity, coordination, and predictable commitment within the government will still be lacking. Without reform, many companies will find themselves in the Valley of Death, unable to bring their ideas from the bench to the bed, and many others, both big and small, will stay on the sidelines.

---

[1] M. Meltzer, et al., "The Economic Impact of Pandemic Influenza in the United States: Priorities for Intervention," *Emerging Infectious Diseases*, 5, no. 5 (September-October 1999): 659.

[2] "Bird Flu Will Cost $800 billion, says World Bank," Times Online, accessed on November 7, 2005 at http://www.timesonline.co.uk/article/0,,25149-1861483,00.html.

Once again, thank-you for the opportunity to testify before the committee today on behalf of BIO. BIO and its member companies are committed to addressing the public health needs of the Nation and look forward to working with this Committee to address these priorities as potential legislation moves forward.

MR. DEAL. Thank you. Mr. Cohen?

MR. COHEN. Thank you. Mr. Chairman and members of the committee, I would like to thank you for giving me the opportunity to speak to you today. I would also like to thank Congresswoman Eshoo for her long history in support of the biotechnology industries, commitment to innovation, job creation, and improvements to our Nation's health. I am the CEO of Cellerant Therapeutics, an early stage biotechnology company based in California, and we are developing novel adult stem cell-based therapies for cancer and genetic blood disorders like sickle cell disease and autoimmune disease. I am here today to talk to you because one of our programs in preclinical development is being developed also for acute radiation syndrome, the principal effect on humans that is likely to result after a nuclear terror attack. We know from our experience at Chernobyl what happens to people who are exposed to lethal doses of radiation, and we are learning through our treatment of people who are being treated for chemotherapy and radiation how to deal with those consequences.

At Cellerant, we are developing a program that is designed to be a bridge therapy for people to control the opportunistic infections and the bleeding implications of radiation exposure, and through support from NIH and our investors, we have developed a novel product that, through peer review research, seems to indicate that it will rescue a substantial number of civilians, that it is stable over a long term in a frozen state, that can be infused by trained medical technicians, and most importantly, that can be administered four to seven days after exposure. If we learn nothing else from the experience with Hurricane Katrina, we know that we need a lot of time to get to people after a mass casualty situation.

I would like to focus specifically on the valley of death, as my colleagues have described the gap between NIH and Project BioShield funding that affects our ability to do process development, commercial scale-up, and clinical trials. The valley of death makes it difficult for us to raise capital and there are three instances of Catch 22 I would like to outline to you. The first is that without human data, you cannot compete for BioShield contracts, but there are no funding mechanisms today to support clinical trials for these agents. The second is many agents like ours have novel manufacturing problems because they are human cell derived, but there is no support for process development in the current legislation. In the third, as is evidenced by the current HHS request proposals, is that you can't get paid until after you produce the drugs and no one in our state can afford to take that financial risk. It makes the program a nonstarter.

The irony of the situation is that many of the incentives in BioShield are for big pharma, but big pharma has little interest in these programs because the markets aren't large enough for them. Small companies are different, and we have different needs. Adding as few as ten people is an agonizing decision for a company of my size, and we can't afford to take the risk without government support. Our investors place a huge premium on our ability to get modest grants from the Federal government that reduces the risk for other investors, it helps us manage our cash, and it provides scientific validation for other investors. For us, big supply contracts are unimpressive because it is not clear we will ever see that money.

There are solutions to the current situation. Specifically, we recommend that the Government find a way to fund the valley of death, the ability to process development, scale-up, and clinical trials that exist between NIH and HHS, and to reduce the risk of the uncertainty associated with some of these very large supply contracts. We think the grant process can be streamlined, as it has in other parts of the Government, and that we can learn how to rely on peer-reviewed published data showing animal efficacy as a basis to fund clinical trials. We can involve the FDA in that process, and they have been terrific in this regard thus far. We can follow some of the examples from DARPA in its ability to provide a commitment to funding, provided milestones are met. And I want to make a point about that.

In our business, a lot of our funding is based on milestones. We get commitments from investors subject to our ability to deliver, and we think the Government should follow that model rather than make us continuously compete for small grants. If we could get up-front commitments subject to milestones, our scientists could focus on doing research instead of writing grant applications. It will allow us to leverage the money from the Government and go out and raise private capital, and it would align our interests with those interests of the country. We are not asking for handouts. There is plenty of capital available for products that have large commercial opportunities. What we are asking for is very modest support to advance programs for the national stockpile.

Business as usual isn't working. The need is urgent, the time is short, and the capacity of our industry is there. We have the resources and we have the talent. What we need is the will to make the required changes to the current system so that we can make rapid progress in fulfilling the Nation's need. Thank you very much.

[The prepared statement of Bruce Cohen follows:]

PREPARED STATEMENT OF BRUCE COHEN, PRESIDENT AND CEO, CELLERANT THERAPEUTICS, INC.

Summary of Prepared Testimony:

Cellerant Therapeutics, Inc. has a preclinical product, CLT-008, that is being developed for civilian applications for the treatment of infections and neutropenia due to radiation therapy and chemotherapy. It also possesses characteristics that make it suitable as a treatment for Acute Radiation Syndrome after a nuclear terror incident:

- **It is a safe, universal, off-the-shelf cell based medicine;**
- **It can be stored frozen in the Strategic National Stockpile for at least 10 years;**
- **It can be deployed to the site of disaster in high density cold storage;**
- **It can be administered up to 7 days post-exposure and still be effective; and**
- **It can be easily administered to patients by intravenous infusion.**

Cellerant has received some modest NIH grant funding to support the development of CLT-008 for biodefense, but has identified three major issues with the current implementation of Bioshield:

(1) Project Bioshield (current law) does not provide specific funding mechanisms for scale up, process development and clinical trials.
(2) The current system does not provide sufficient incentives for small, private companies and seems to favor large corporations.
(3) Current law does not encourage innovation.

Cellerant suggests the following solutions:

(1) Authorize funding, through an existing or new agency, to address pre-clinical scale up and cost reduction: the current "Valley of Death" for Bioshield product development.
(2) Authorize a new or existing agency to fund human safety trials for countermeasures being developed for Bioshield.
(3) Establish an improved formal mechanism, other than SBIR, for funding small companies engaged in biodefense research and product development.

Good afternoon and thank you for the opportunity to testify before the Subcommittee today. My name is Bruce Cohen, and I am the President and Chief Executive Officer of Cellerant Therapeutics, Inc., a clinical stage biotechnology company developing adult stem cell based therapies for cancer, genetic blood disorders and autoimmune disease. I am presenting this testimony because one of our pre-clinical products is also being developed as a universal counter-measure to improve survival and treat Acute Radiation Syndrome resulting from a nuclear terror incident. While the devastation of such an attack is difficult to contemplate, it is incumbent upon us to develop strategies that can rescue as many victims as we possibly can.

Radiation is an important therapy in the treatment of various cancers. Doses of chemotherapy and radiation that damage the blood-forming and gastrointestinal systems are frequently employed in the treatment of cancers or preparation for hematopoietic cell transplantation. Our product, CLT-008, is a cultured myeloid progenitor cell product that we have developed to address a pressing need in medicine – patients with compromised immune systems as a result of chemotherapy and radiation treatments. Despite advances in medical care, these patients are highly vulnerable to infections and internal bleeding with a significant risk of mortality.

From a medical perspective, these patients are very much like those we would encounter in the aftermath of a nuclear terror incident such as an attack on a nuclear power plant or the detonation of a nuclear weapon smuggled in a container vessel. Much of what we know about the impact of radiation on civilian populations is based on our experience at Chernobyl. Depending upon the dose of radiation to which a person is exposed, a variety of medical problems can ensue with serious organ involvement, described generally as Acute Radiation Syndrome, the precise manifestations of which will be highly variable and dependent on the nature of the exposure. The most therapeutically addressable manifestation of ARS is known as hematopoietic syndrome, in which the blood-forming and immune system is damaged. Following a nuclear terror incident, civilians and first responders would receive doses of radiation that would profoundly damage their blood-forming and immune systems to the extent that they would not be able to resist common infections or recover from internal bleeding. Even temporary failure of the blood-forming and immune system without adequate medical support can be lethal, especially in a mass casualty setting.

Our extensive studies in preclinical animal models of lethal irradiation have been published in peer-reviewed scientific journals and predict that our product, CLT-008, will be capable of rescuing a significant number of victims of nuclear terror. Our studies suggest that CLT-008 protects against lethal infections and can be administered 4-7 days after radiation exposure. Decades of clinical experience in cell cryopreservation and infusion predict that our product will be stable in frozen vials for as long as 10 years, making it suitable for inclusion in the Strategic National Stockpile. CLT-008 can be infused by any medical technician trained in the administration of intravenous infusions. Our product offers the potential for a bridging therapy, providing victims with temporary immune competence for 30-45 days, allowing them time to seek more durable treatments when the situation becomes more stable.

No other pharmaceutical product, whether approved or in development, is able to permanently or temporarily reconstitute the immune system to the degree necessary to rescue large numbers of civilians, first responders, or warfighters. Of the limited number of products proposed, most would have to be given before or immediately after exposure, something that is unlikely to be practical in the event of a catastrophic nuclear terror incident. Most medical experts agree that orally-available drugs are unlikely to be effective in restoring an immune system which has suffered profound damage from radiation. Cell-based medicines, like the one we have under development, hold the promise of being able to rescue large numbers of otherwise lethally irradiated victims, in a timely manner and with the limited medical capabilities that are likely to be available in the aftermath of a nuclear terror event.

Our experience with the U.S. Government in developing this product as a countermeasure to nuclear terror has been mixed. We have been awarded modestly sized, peer-reviewed research grants from the NIH. However, we have been frustrated by the limitations of the current system in its ability to support the next stage of development – confirmation of safety and efficacy in humans. I would like to outline the limitations of the current system and suggest some alternatives.

(1) Project Bioshield (current law) does not provide specific funding mechanisms for scale up, process development and clinical trials.

While it is technically possible under existing law for the NIH to fund projects related to commercial scale-up, process development aimed at cost-reduction, and the initiation of human clinical trials, grant mechanisms to support this activity for private companies do not exist or are extremely limited in scope. The NIH peer-review grant process has been an extraordinary contributor to the advancement of science and medicine in the U.S., but it has not focused on translating those discoveries toward commercial applications in the private sector. For most medical products, this is appropriate, as the pharmaceutical industry, venture capital community and public investors have been able to make the necessary investments that have made the U.S. the world's leader in biotechnology. However, those sources of capital are not available for the development of medical products whose primary customer is the U.S. Government through Project Bioshield acquisition. Typical private investors will not assume the risk of doing business with the Government, specifically making a large investment in research without a firm commitment to make the contemplated purchase.

Since the current Bioshield program does not allow the Government to enter into contracts with companies until they have shown human safety and have a defined, and cost-effective manufacturing process, companies like Cellerant find themselves in the Valley of Death. That is, we do not have adequate financial resources to move our pre-clinical programs aggressively into human clinical trials, but without the results of those trials, we cannot compete for contracts under Project Bioshield. In addition, to the extent we are developing novel agents that have not previously been manufactured, we are likely to have production economics that will make the purchase contract unattractive, either from the Government's perspective of total cost or the company's perspective of generating an adequate return on investor capital.

This Valley of Death funding gap means that, in our case, we have had to slow development of our product in accordance with our ability to raise venture capital based on a non-Government application of our technology. That funding is available, but it takes an enormous amount of time and effort, and our investors are not prepared to have us use their capital for a program whose financing is beyond the control of the commercial pharmaceutical market.

(2) The current system does not provide sufficient incentives for small, private companies and seems to favor large corporations.

The current Bioshield program is biased toward the purchase of products which have been developed and approved for other reasons and which are being re-directed toward biodefense countermeasures. For example, the currently pending Bioshield nuclear countermeasure acquisition offer from HHS requires that eligible contractors manufacture a minimum number of doses prior to being paid by the Government. That is practical for a product which already has a defined commercial market, since the inventory could be used for other purposes in the event the Government decides not to complete the purchase. For an innovative product like ours, which has higher manufacturing costs, the risk of producing a large lot with no guaranteed buyer is unacceptable. That risk may well be borne by a larger company with greater capital resources, but it discourages small companies from competing.

The irony of the current system that seems to favor large companies is this: for most large pharmaceutical companies, the economics and market potential associated with producing biodefense products do not justify the commitment of significant resources, because their investors are expecting the development of blockbuster products and do not value the financial impact of a Government contract. For emerging biotech companies, what appears to be a relatively small market to a larger company may well be considered a substantial business opportunity. In addition, investors in biotech companies highly value the award of even a modestly sized contract because it is significant relative to the company's cash requirements and because it is seen as a form of scientific validation. Small companies are also more efficient in developing innovative new medical therapies, particularly for specialty applications.

(3) Current law does not encourage innovation.

Innovation comes from taking a fresh look at a problem and leads to the development of novel entities. The current process unfortunately encourages derivative development, i.e., finding new uses for old inventions. Thus, it becomes quite practical for a company to identify a new indication for an established drug (e.g., Ciprofloxacin as a treatment for anthrax), but the current rules do not encourage small, innovative companies to challenge current thinking, create novel paradigms, and make therapeutic breakthroughs.

In our domain, adult-derived cell therapies, we have a very different approach to the development of medicines. Our products are based on human cells. The science behind our approach has been translated into clinical practice for more than 40 years with relatively low risk for toxicity. However, cell-based therapies uniformly incur high manufacturing costs since they are derived from human source material and must be processed in controlled environments. We do not enjoy conventional pharmaceutical economics where the cost of the product itself is relatively modest compared to the cost of research and development. Both (a) the inability of the Government to fund research related to cost-reducing the manufacture of cellular medicines and (b) the procurement policies related to the need to produce numbers of doses prior to getting paid make it very difficult for innovative approaches to succeed. Successful translation of scientific innovations to protect us from the medical consequences of nuclear attack requires innovation in the funding mechanisms.

We believe that there are a number of solutions to the problems that we and others have encountered.

(1) The first solution would be to specifically authorize funding to address the Valley of Death. The Government, either through a new agency, the NIH, or HHS/Bioshield, should be able to enter into non-competitive contracts for the achievement of very specific tasks, relating to the nation's priorities in national defense, for pre-clinical scale up for promising products that have demonstrated potential based on peer-reviewed animal experiments. Competitive review is appropriate for early stage work, where it is not possible to determine the probability of success except with highly trained peer reviewers. However, the rigor of a well established academic and private sector peer-review process, as evidenced by publications in major journals or presentation at recognized national meetings, can be used to accelerate programs which have already demonstrated scientific and clinical merit. There is no need to delay the award of contracts for the achievement of very specific purposes by insisting on a prolonged scientific competition.

(2) The second solution would be to direct, not simply authorize, a new or existing agency to fund human safety trials for products being developed as priority biodefense countermeasures, particularly nuclear countermeasures. While such authority technically exists within current authorities throughout HHS and DOD, a Congressional mandate to address this key element of the Valley of Death would encourage innovation and ensure the participation of smaller companies. The Government could easily put into place the necessary controls and require the concurrence of the FDA as to the readiness of the product for human trials, a rigorous process that has served the industry and our country quite well.

(3) The third solution would be to establish an improved formal mechanism for funding small companies engaged in biodefense research and product development. The limitations with the current SBIR program, including the relatively low level of funding provided in the first year and the modest levels provided in additional years, make this program an inefficient and time-consuming mechanism for funding research to address urgent and potentially catastrophic terror events. One such

> option would be to provide promising technologies with multi-year commitments that would be subject to the completion of specific milestones, in much the same way as private investors commit capital contingent on technological achievements being met. This would make the grant programs more attractive because the promise of milestone-driven funding would then justify the expense and time associated with grant preparation, provided, of course, that the technology proved to be valuable.

Throughout the country, there are academic and commercial enterprises that have access to extraordinarily talented people and ideas. A modest investment by the Government, coupled with the relaxation of a few counter-productive restrictions would unleash this capacity and provide the nation with the ability to respond to an event of unimaginable consequences.

Thank you again for the opportunity to testify today. I would be pleased to answer any questions you may have.

MR. DEAL. Thank you. And Dr. Wright?

DR. WRIGHT. Thank you, Mr. Chairman. For the record, it is Dr. Wright. Mr. Chairman, members of the committee, I welcome the opportunity to testify on behalf of the Alliance for Biosecurity and commend this committee for its focus on the vital issues of biosecurity and the Project BioShield legislation. I am David Wright, Co-Chair of the Alliance for Biosecurity, President and CEO of PharmAthene, a biotech company focusing totally on biodefense. The Alliance for Biosecurity is a consortium of 12 biotechnology and pharmaceutical companies committed to promoting a new era in the prevention and treatment of severe infectious diseases, particularly those that present global security challenges, through innovative and accelerated research and development and through production of countermeasures.

The majority of medicines and vaccines needed to protect our citizens during attack does not now exist, and creating a robust biodefense infrastructure and pipeline of countermeasures simply cannot be accomplished overnight. The modest number of companies now working on biodefense projects are increasingly unlikely to continue to invest in this challenging area, absent strong new biodefense legislation that supports and facilitates countermeasure development and production for our strategic national stockpile. For these reasons, we urge you to support passage of focused and strategic biodefense legislation this year.

On behalf of the Alliance, I would like to discuss three key areas. First, clarity in establishing a central authority is necessary. Currently, there is a littering away of agencies and overlapping conflicting authorities over biosecurity. A biodefense structure that streamlines decision-making and identifies a clear point of accountability within the Government is urgently needed. The Alliance supports a restructuring of the current process that creates a clearly identified centralized biodefense authority. The centralized authority should coordinate with NIH to identify and prioritize early countermeasure development, fund advanced development of promising countermeasures, the period which has been referred to here as the valley of death, and oversee all strategic national stockpile procurement.

Second, building a partnership between the Government and industry is a critical component to the success of Project BioShield. The development of bioterror countermeasures is a very risky endeavor, even more risky, in fact, than traditional pharmaceutical development for several reasons. There is only one customer, the U.S. Government. Procurement funds are limited, and only one or a limited number of products per category will actually be purchased. It is therefore crucial that DHHS outline publicly its priorities across all countermeasure targets and estimated timelines for procurement. We urge DHHS to actively communicate with companies and to include industry thoroughly and often in the process.

Finally, a real commitment to fund biosecurity is paramount. The current reserve fund of $5.6 billion established under Project BioShield is insufficient to address all but a few of the pressing biological threats. Industry is looking to Congress and the Administration to signal that biosecurity preparedness is a national security priority justifying a considerable commitment by industry. In order to do this, a major paradigm shift is needed in how our Nation thinks about defense against emerging infectious diseases that have the potential to be significant and destabilizing. We urge this committee to champion a level of funding for countermeasure development that is commensurate with the magnitude of the national security threat and corresponding requirements. Sufficient, sustained funding is absolutely critical to the success of Project BioShield.

In summary, developing a central authority for biosecurity, improving cooperation and communication between the Government and industry by forming a real partnership, and committing the necessary funding to make meaningful scientific and commercial progress are each practical recommendations for improvement. On behalf of the Alliance for Biosecurity and its member companies, I respectfully submit these recommendations for your consideration. Thank you.

[The prepared statement of Dr. David P. Wright follows:]

PREPARED STATEMENT OF DR. DAVID P. WRIGHT, PRESIDENT AND CEO, PHARMATHENE, ON BEHALF OF ALLIANCE FOR BIOSECURITY

Mr. Chairman, Members of the Subcommittee: I welcome the opportunity to testify before you today on behalf of the Alliance for Biosecurity and commend this committee for its focus on the vital issue of biodefense and Project BioShield legislation.

I am David Wright, Co-Chair of the Alliance for Biosecurity and President and Chief Executive Officer of PharmAthene, a biotechnology company specializing in the development and commercialization of biological and chemical defense countermeasures. The Alliance for Biosecurity is a consortium that includes the Center for Biosecurity of the University of Pittsburgh Medical Center and 12 biotechnology and pharmaceutical companies committed to promoting a new era in the prevention and treatment of severe infectious diseases -- particularly those that present global security challenges -- through innovative and accelerated research, development, and production of countermeasures. The Alliance includes companies focused on infectious disease like GlaxoSmithKline, Chiron, and Pfizer. Other member companies, such as Acambis, VaxGen, and BioPort have been successful in garnering contracts under Project BioShield and its precursor programs, while members like PharmAthene and other Alliance companies are poised to compete for new procurement contracts. We believe that based on this considerable collective experience, the Alliance is well positioned to address lessons learned from current implementation of Project BioShield and assist in the development of solutions to improve the program going forward. A list of our members appears at the conclusion of this testimony.

Project BioShield was a critical first step in demonstrating the government's commitment to biodefense. The Alliance applauds the commitment demonstrated by Congress towards this initiative as well as the hard work undertaken by government officials to implement a complex new program. Now that the foundation has been laid, the Alliance believes that more targeted action, expanded public/private partnerships, and clear and accountable leadership is needed to provide the support and incentives necessary to develop the robust biodefense industry as envisioned in the original BioShield legislation. The majority of medicines and vaccines needed to protect our citizens during an attack do not now exist, and creating a robust biodefense infrastructure and pipeline of countermeasures simply cannot be accomplished overnight. The modest number of companies now working on biodefense projects are increasingly unlikely to continue to invest in this challenging area absent strong new biodefense legislation that supports and facilitates countermeasure development and production for our nation's Strategic National Stockpile. For these reasons, in considering the reauthorization of certain provisions under the current Project BioShield Act, we urge you to support passage of focused and strategic improvements to this critical biodefense legislation this year.

On behalf of the Alliance, I would like to discuss three key areas, which, if addressed, could significantly advance the biodefense market and the availability of critical countermeasures to protect the American people.

- **Clarity in Establishing a Central Authority**

The first issue involves clarifying who is in charge and ensuring that the responsible Government agencies understand the intricacies and challenges of drug development. Such a critical knowledge base should inform the Government's research, development and procurement decisions. Currently, there is a bewildering array of agencies with overlapping and conflicting authority over biosecurity. A biodefense structure that streamlines decision-making and identifies a clear point of accountability within the government is urgently needed. The Alliance supports a restructuring of the current process that creates a clearly identified centralized biodefense authority. The centralized authority should coordinate with NIH to identify and prioritize early countermeasure development, fund advanced development of promising countermeasures (the period sometimes referred to as the "valley of death") and oversee all SNS procurement. This central authority could also coordinate closely with DHS on the threat assessments. It is absolutely critical that the new central authority be led and staffed by people who are knowledgeable about commercial drug development, including medicine and vaccine research and development, clinical testing, and manufacturing processes. A major influx of personnel with expertise and experience in drug development would greatly improve the central authority's ability to work quickly and efficiently with industry to acquire needed countermeasures for our nation's stockpile. Ideally, such people would also have experience with biodefense drug development and some experience with non-clinical testing under the FDA's "Animal Rule".

These changes could be accomplished through, for instance, the establishment of the proposed Biomedical Advanced Research and Development Agency (BARDA) in Senate bill 1873 if it were explicitly given clear authority, or through other administrative mechanisms.

In March, Secretary Leavitt indicated in testimony before the Senate his intention to restructure the Office of Public Health Emergency Preparedness to improve the efficiency of development and procurement of countermeasures. He expressed a willingness to work with Congress on these changes and we strongly desire and hope he will reach out to industry as well. I emphasize that we will only be successful in this endeavor if government and industry work together in partnership. This brings me to my second recommendation:

- **Building a Partnership Between Government and Industry**

This is another critical component to revitalizing Project BioShield. The development of bioterror countermeasures is a very risky endeavor, more risky in fact than traditional pharmaceutical development for several reasons: there is only one customer – the US government, procurement funds are limited and only one, or a limited number of products per category will actually be purchased. It is, therefore, crucial that DHHS work with industry to communicate in a transparent fashion its priorities across all countermeasure targets, estimated timelines for procurement, and expected procurement quantities. We urge DHHS to actively communicate with companies and to include industry early and often in the process. We wish to closely partner with government to accomplish our nation's biodefense goals. The Alliance believes that improved information sharing and partnering between the US government and industry would result in more companies entering this market and better products that meet the government's specifications. For example, the new centralized authority could improve communication with industry by:

- *Instituting a consistent update mechanism (for example with a list serve or website) to alert industry to key activities – issuance of a new Material Threat Assessment or Determination, or an upcoming RFI, RFP or other notice.*
- *Holding an annual or biannual Advance Planning Briefing* to share information on current programs, identify new areas of interest, and seek industry partners. DOD does this routinely.
- *Allowing industry to present data on their technologies to inter-agency working groups.* The decision-making process for bioterror products is fragmented and involves many different agencies and departments. DHHS should provide an opportunity for companies with promising technologies to regularly present products to the group and engage in a discussion with working group members. These types of interactions would help industry to develop products that better meet the government's needs.
- *Allowing industry access to data on relevant animal models.* Initiating research with the appropriate animal model(s) is a key factor in the success of drug development. It is also critical in the acceptance of company data by the FDA. Unfortunately, there is no direct mechanism to establish communication/relationships with US government scientists. Allowing communication between US government resources and companies developing products in this area will provide an opportunity for industry to more consistently design the animal studies, which are critical in determining efficacy.

- *Clearly identifying a lead/group/point of contact with specific responsibility for interfacing with industry on a daily basis.* Maintaining good relations and facilitating clear communications with an active and engaged industrial base is critical for the success of the BioShield program, now and in the future.

- **Commitment to Fund Biosecurity**

The final point I would like to address today focuses on the U.S. government's commitment to fund biosecurity. The current reserve fund of $5.6 billion established under Project BioShield, to be used over a 10-year period, is insufficient to address all but a few of the most pressing biological threats. Potential public health disasters caused by exposure to known and emerging pathogens must be viewed as a pressing national security issue. We know that the raw materials and scientific knowledge necessary to develop bioweapons are widely available. The scale of social and economic disruption that would be caused by a bioterror attack could be unlike anything in recent US history – even the aftermath of Hurricane Katrina. Yet, the current levels of funding for biosecurity do not match the threat. Further, discussions among Alliance companies and DHHS officials indicate that after only two years into the BioShield program, the paucity of funding and limitations on how much can be spent annually is already adversely affecting the willingness or perceived ability of government staff to make procurement commitments and issue RFPs.

Industry is looking to Congress and the Administration to signal that biosecurity preparedness is a national security priority justifying a considerable commitment by the government. In order to do this, a major paradigm shift is needed in how our nation thinks about defense against bioterrorism and, at the same time, defense against emerging infectious diseases that have the potential to be significantly destabilizing.

We urge this committee to champion a level of funding for countermeasure development that is commensurate with the magnitude of the national security threat and corresponding requirements. Sufficient, sustained funding is absolutely critical to the success of Project BioShield. Currently, the average chance for a drug that enters Phase I clinical trials to eventually be approved is about 8 percent; for cancer drugs, it is about 5 percent. For companies to face similar odds in developing biodefense countermeasures, it is critical for them and their investors to feel confident that the government has defined and will support a reliable market for the procurement of the countermeasures.

If additional direct funding cannot at this point be provided, we urge Congress to consider in biodefense legislation indirect incentives that could greatly increase the number of companies prepared to invest in countermeasure development. Bioterrorism countermeasures are much like drugs intended for diseases that afflict very few people (so-called "orphan" drugs), in that neither class of medicine has a sufficient market to adequately encourage development. Congress recognized that market-based incentives such as additional marketing exclusivity could provide an efficient means of encouraging drug development when it enacted the Orphan Drugs Act, and that Act has been successful in encouraging the development of new drugs for orphan diseases. In a similar way, other forms of incentives could be explored as a means of encouraging the development of bioterrorism countermeasures. The Alliance is available to dialogue with the Subcommittee to explore such options.

In summary, if we wish to create and maintain a biodefense industry that fosters innovation and investment by the private sector, then we must heed the lessons learned from current implementation and apply new solutions to the challenges posed by such a marketplace. Developing a central authority for biosecurity, improving co-operation and communication between government and industry by forming a real partnership, and committing the necessary funding to make meaningful progress, are each practical recommendations for improvement. On behalf of the Alliance for Biosecurity and its members, I respectfully submit these recommendations for your consideration.

<u>Members of the Alliance for Biosecurity:</u>
Acambis, Inc.
Caprion Pharmaceuticals, Inc.
Center for Biosecurity of the University of Pittsburgh Medical Center
Chiron Corporation
DOR BioPharma, Inc.
Dynport Vaccines Co., LLC, a CSC company
Emergent BioSolutions
GlaxoSmithKline
Human Genome Sciences, Inc.
Idenix Pharmaceuticals, Inc.
Pfizer Inc.
PharmAthene
VaxGen, Inc.

MR. DEAL. Thank you. Dr. Blaser?

DR. BLASER. Mr. Chairman and committee members, thank you for inviting the Infectious Diseases Society of America to present our views. I am Martin Blaser, President of the IDSA and Chair of Medicine and Professor of Microbiology at the New York University School of Medicine.

IDSA is a national medical society representing 8,000 infectious disease physicians and scientists. Today, we highlight the critical need for new drugs, vaccines, and diagnostics to detect, prevent, and treat naturally occurring infectious disease agents. In particular, we highlight our patients' need for new antibiotics to treat resistant bacterial infections as this pipeline is rapidly drying up. As this subcommittee considers reauthorization of the BioShield Act, IDSA urges you to strengthen the emphasis on products intended to be used against naturally occurring infectious diseases, including infections resistant to antibiotics. We ask that you consider adding several new incentives to BioShield to spur the development of infectious disease products. BioShield guarantees a market, but to develop antibiotics for resistant organisms, we need broader incentives.

In its 2003 report on the BioShield Act, the Energy and Commerce Committee linked natural conditions, including antimicrobial resistance in dangerous viruses, to natural security concerns. The report stated, advancing the discovery of new antimicrobial agents to treat resistant organisms may well pay dividends for both national security and public health. We agree. In 2004, IDSA issued a report entitled "Bad Bugs, No Drugs, As Antibiotic Discovery Stagnates, A Public Health Crisis Brews." Copies of that report are available here today. Our report highlights that drug companies are withdrawing from antibiotic R and D. As a result, the pharmaceutical pipeline simply is not keeping pace with drug-resistant bacterial infections. Antibiotics have saved millions of lives for more than 60 years, however, without new R and D, we may soon be back in the dark ages of medicine. Imagine a world without antibiotics; but that is where we are heading. Companies have lost interest because antibiotics simply are not as profitable as drugs that treat chronic conditions.

Most antibiotics are used for short durations and face restrictive uses to avoid the development of resistance. Antibiotic-resistant infections have created a silent epidemic in communities and hospitals across the country. Methicillin staph aureus is crippling and killing a growing number of athletes, children, and military recruits. Resistant bacteria can strike anyone; the young, the old, the healthy, and the infirm. Resistant pathogens lead to higher healthcare costs in part because they require extended hospital stays. The hospital care earlier this year for Bryce Smith, a 14-month-old toddler from San Diego, cost more than $800,000. The total cost of antimicrobial resistance to the U.S. healthcare system was about $5 billion in 1998, according to the Institute of Medicine. It is believed that true costs far exceed that amount today, since resistance is increasing. Importantly, since 1998, FDA has approved only 13 new antibiotics, only two of which are truly novel. In 2002, among 89 new medicines emerging on the market, none was an antibiotic.

In addition to antibiotics, vaccines and diagnostics are needed across the spectrum of infectious disease medicines, including to address the growing threat of pandemic flu. The impact of an influenza pandemic cannot be overstated. The CDC estimates that between 100,000 and 250,000 U.S. deaths would result from a mild pandemic, and that 900,000 to two million Americans will die from a virus as bad as the 1918 virus. Therefore, robust industry R and D programs are urgently needed across the spectrum of infectious disease medicine, but market forces alone are not sufficient. This is why we need the Infectious Disease Research and Development Act, a bipartisan bill introduced by Representative Cubin last year. IDSA strongly endorses this bill and is particularly grateful to Representative Cubin's leadership. We encourage the committee to consider this bill as it moves forward to reauthorize Project BioShield.

The Cubin Bill will establish a commission to identify the most dangerous infectious disease pathogens and their associated diseases. Based on the commission's recommendations, several incentives would be used to spur development of new antibiotics, antivirals, diagnostic tests, and vaccines. Until the commission gets up and running, the incentives outlined would be available immediately to spur products to use against MRSA, acinetobacter, a bacteria that has caused wound infections and hospitalized patients, and wounds in U.S. soldiers in Iraq, and against influenza. The Cubin Bill includes a number of incentives for qualified products, including full restoration of patent terms to account for the time lost during FDA review; and a tax credit for facilities used to manufacture, distribute and for R and D, allowing manufacturers to take a tax credit on research expenses.

We also encourage the subcommittee to consider three other incentives: providing an FDA priority review voucher to companies that obtains an approval for a qualified product; extending the patent term on qualified products for two years or even six months. We recommend strengthening CDC's Antimicrobial Program by doubling its budget in fiscal year 2007 to $50 million so it can better lead our Nation's response to antimicrobial resistance.

In conclusion, we cannot take a business-as-usual approach. The bad bugs are not waiting and neither should we. The IDSA appreciates the opportunity to testify today and to work with your committee. Thank you.

[The prepared statement of Dr. Martin Blaser follows:]

PREPARED STATEMENT OF DR. MARTIN BLASER, PRESIDENT, INFECTIOUS DISEASES SOCIETY OF AMERICA

Chairman Deal, Ranking Member Brown and Members of the Subcommittee, thank you for inviting the Infectious Diseases Society of America (IDSA) to present our views on how best to strengthen Project Bioshield as the Subcommittee considers its reauthorization. I am Dr. Martin J. Blaser, President of IDSA and a Frederick H. King Professor and Chair of the Department of Medicine, and Professor of Microbiology at NYU School of Medicine.

IDSA represents 8,000 physicians and scientists devoted to patient care, education, research, prevention, and community health planning in infectious diseases. Our members care for patients of all ages with serious infections, including antibiotic-resistant bacterial infections, meningitis, pneumonia, tuberculosis, food poisoning, HIV/AIDS, and those with cancer or transplants who have life-threatening infections caused by unusual microorganisms, as well as emerging infections like severe acute respiratory syndrome (SARS). Housed within IDSA is the HIV Medicine Association (HIVMA), which represents more than 3,200 physicians working on the frontline of the HIV/AIDS pandemic. HIVMA members conduct research, implement prevention programs, and provide clinical services to individuals that are infected with HIV/AIDS. Together, IDSA and HIVMA are the principal organizations representing infectious diseases and HIV physicians in the United States.

I am testifying today on behalf of IDSA to highlight the critical need for new drugs, vaccines and diagnostics to treat, prevent and detect infectious diseases agents. As Members of the Subcommittee move forward to consider the reauthorization of the Project Bioshield Act, IDSA urges you to extend the statutes' scope beyond products intended to address bioterrorism-related pathogens and apply current incentives to products to be used against naturally occurring infectious diseases, including antimicrobial resistant infections. We also ask that you add several new provisions to Bioshield that will help to eliminate disincentives and to spur infectious diseases product development both related to naturally occurring infections and biodefense.

Members of the Energy and Commerce Committee have shown that they understand the connection between naturally occurring infections and bioterrorism and understand our nation's vulnerability. In its 2003 Committee report on the Project Bioshield Act, the Committee linked *natural conditions*, including antimicrobial resistance and dangerous viruses, to national security concerns. The Report stated "advancing the discovery of new antimicrobial drugs to treat resistant organisms ... may well pay dividends for both national security and public health."

IDSA believes that there is an inextricably linked, synergistic relationship between the research and development (R&D) needed to protect against both natural occurring infections and bioterrorism agents. Research in both areas seeks to understand how these organisms cause disease, the immune system response to these pathogens, the development of drug resistance, and how antibiodies and medicines protect against them. Moreover, antibiotic resistant organisms that currently threaten Americans in hospitals and communities can have future national and global security implications. Virtually all of the antibiotic-resistant pathogens that exist naturally today can be bio-engineered through forced mutation or cloning. Expanding the government's product development priorities to include naturally occurring infections will enhance the research needed to develop bioterrorism countermeasures and vice versa.

Background

On July 21, 2004, the same day that President Bush signed "The Project Bioshield Act", IDSA issued its landmark report entitled, *Bad Bugs, No Drugs, As Antibiotic Discovery Stagnates, A Public Health Crisis Brews.* Copies of that report are available here today. Our report calls attention to a serious public health problem—at the same time that emerging infections and antibiotic resistance are increasing, drug companies are withdrawing from antiinfective R&D. IDSA is particularly concerned about antibiotic R&D, an area in which many pharmaceutical and biotechnology companies have shown the least commitment in recent years, either withdrawing totally or seriously downsizing their dedicated resources and staff.

Let me be very clear from the start: IDSA is here today on behalf of patients. We are not here at the request of the pharmaceutical or biotechnology industries nor is our *Bad Bugs, No Drugs* advocacy campaign financed in any way by industry. Infectious diseases (ID) and HIV physicians on the frontline of patient care see patients every day who face lengthy and expensive hospitalizations, painful courses of treatment and even death because of drug-resistant and other infections. We are here because our patients desperately need new weapons to protect them against these diseases.

Why Policymakers Should be Concerned

Policymakers have recognized the urgent need to spur biodefense R&D, which led to the establishment of Project Bioshield. While concern about bioterrorism is appropriate, it is important to keep things in perspective. Not one American has died from bioterrorism since President Bush first announced Project Bioshield in February of 2003, but drug-resistant bacterial and other infections have killed hundreds of thousands of Americans in hospitals and communities across the United States and millions of people across the world during that same short period of time.

Here are some surprising facts about the impact of drug-resistant bacterial infections in the United States:

- Antimicrobial resistant infections have created a "silent epidemic" in communities and hospitals across the country—methicillin-resistant staphylococcus aureus (MRSA), for example, is crippling and killing a growing number of athletes, children, military recruits, and prisoners.
- Infections caused by resistant bacteria can strike anyone—the young and the old, the healthy and the chronically ill. Theresa Drew recently shared the story of her son, Ricky Lannetti, with congressional staff. Ricky, a healthy and strong 21-year old college football player from Philadelphia, Pennsylvania

succumbed to an MRSA infection in December 2003. Ricky's story is just the tip of the iceberg.

- About 2 million people acquire bacterial infections in U.S. hospitals each year, and 90,000 die as a result. About 70 percent of those infections are resistant to at least one drug. Community-acquired resistant infections also are on the rise. The trends toward increasing drug resistance in both hospitals and communities show no sign of abating.
- Resistant pathogens lead to higher health care costs because they often require more expensive drugs and extended hospital stays. The hospital care for Bryce Smith, a 14-month old toddler from San Diego, cost more than $800,000 in the beginning months of 2006. The total cost of antimicrobial resistance to the U.S. health care system was nearly $5 billion in 1998, according to the Institute of Medicine (IOM). It is believed true costs far exceed that amount today.

What policymakers should know about pandemic influenza:

- The impact of an influenza pandemic cannot be overstated. The Centers for Disease Control and Prevention (CDC) estimates that between 100,000-250,000 U.S. deaths would result from a "mild" pandemic and 900,000–2 million Americans will die from a virus as deadly as the 1918 virus.
- The Congressional Budget Office estimated that a pandemic could cost $675 billion and decrease the real gross domestic product (GDP) by five percent.
- H5N1 avian influenza has spread rapidly in the past few months to more than 40 countries in Asia, Africa, the Middle East and Europe. Experts agree that it is only a matter of time before it appears among birds in North America.
- H5N1 virus is showing continued evolution, and has infected an increasing variety of mammals. A moderate number of human cases continue with a high death rate. Fortunately, the virus is not yet capable of easily spreading from person to person; should this happen, a dramatic pandemic will occur.
- Despite the increased attention and progress that has been made in preparing for an influenza pandemic, the Institute of Medicine and virtually all experts conclude that the United States is woefully unprepared to sufficiently respond to pandemic flu and many gaps and challenges remain.
- Moreover, seasonal influenza accounts for 36,000 deaths and more than 200,000 hospitalizations in the United States and 250,000 to 500,000 deaths globally each year.

Here are some important facts about other infectious diseases:

- Three of the biggest killers—HIV, tuberculosis (TB) and malaria—account for nearly 40 percent of deaths caused by infectious diseases (5.6 million deaths in 2002).
- Diarrheal diseases and respiratory infections are equally as deadly, accounting for 5.7 million deaths in 2002.
- More than three-dozen new infectious diseases have been identified since the 1970s that have impacted the United States and more vulnerable countries, including HIV/AIDS, SARS, West Nile virus, Lyme disease, hepatitis C, a new form of cholera, waterborne disease due to *Cryptosporidium*, foodborne disease caused by *E. coli* 0157:H7, and a plethora of neglected diseases that primarily affect patients in the developing world.

The Product Pipeline is Drying Up

Infectious diseases are the second leading cause of death in the world and, by far, the leading cause of premature death and disability. Unfortunately, many of these diseases have no treatment except for supportive care. New medicines and diagnostics are desperately needed across all areas of infectious diseases medicine.

Of particular concern, the pipeline of new antibiotics is drying up. Major pharmaceutical companies are losing interest in the antibiotics market because these drugs simply are not as profitable as drugs that treat chronic, life-long conditions and lifestyle issues. The pharmaceutical pipeline is not keeping pace with drug-resistant bacterial infections, so-called "superbugs." Antibiotics, like other antimicrobial drugs, have saved millions of lives and eased patients' suffering. The withdrawal of companies from antibiotic R&D is a frightening twist to the antibiotic resistance problem and, we believe, one that has not received adequate attention from federal policymakers.

A recent analysis published in the journal *Clinical Infectious Diseases* found only five new antibiotics in the R&D pipeline out of more than 506 drugs in development. The authors evaluated the websites or 2002 annual reports of 15 major pharmaceutical companies with a track record in antibiotic development and seven major biotechnology companies. Their analysis revealed four new antibiotics being developed by pharmaceutical companies, and only one antibiotic being developed by a biotech company. By comparison, the analysis found that the pharmaceutical companies were developing 67 new drugs for cancer, 33 for inflammation/pain, 34 for metabolic/endocrine disorders, and 32 for pulmonary disease. The biotech companies were developing 24 drugs for inflammation/immunomodulators, 14 drugs for metabolic/endocrine disorders, and 13 for cancer.

The end result of the decline in antibiotic discovery research is that the Food and Drug Administration (FDA) is approving few new antibiotics. Since 1998, only 13 new antibiotics have been approved, two of which are truly novel—i.e., defined as having a new target of action, with no cross-resistance with other antibiotics. In 2002, among 89 new medicines emerging on the market, none was an antibiotic.

The Institute of Medicine's (IOM) 2003 report on microbial threats reinforces the point, noting that although at first glance the situation with respect to antibiotics currently in clinical development looks encouraging, not one *new class* of antibiotics is in late-stage development. "Rather these 'new' antibiotics belong to existing classes, including macrolides and quinolones, that have been used to treat humans for years," IOM said.

Unfortunately, both the public and private sectors appear to have been lulled into a false sense of security based on past successes. The potential crisis at hand is the result of a marked decrease in industry R&D, government inaction, and the increasing prevalence of resistant bacteria.

IDSA has investigated the decline in new antibiotic R&D for more than three years, interviewing stakeholders from all sectors. We have met with officials from FDA, the National Institute of Allergy and Infectious Diseases (NIAID), CDC, congressional members and staff, executives from leading pharmaceutical and biotechnology companies, representatives from public-private partnerships that are focused on infectious diseases-related product development, patients, and other stakeholders.

Based on our investigation, IDSA is convinced that the pharmaceutical and biotechnology industries are clearly best situated to take the lead in developing new antibiotics needed to treat bacterial diseases. They are the only player with a track record of success. Consequently, industry action must become the central focus of an innovative federal public health effort designed to stimulate antibiotic R&D.

Some people have placed the blame for the decline in R&D on the pharmaceutical industry, saying that companies should act responsibly and ensure that new drugs and vaccines are available as needed. The pharmaceutical industry supports many good works *pro bono*. Some examples include Merck & Co.'s efforts related to River

Blindness; efforts by Bristol-Myers Squibb, Pfizer, and other drug companies related to global AIDS; and GlaxoSmithKline's malaria and AstraZeneca's TB drug discovery initiatives. Nevertheless, companies are responsible to their shareholders and cannot alter their fundamental business strategies in ways that would place their bottom lines at risk.

Drug and vaccine R&D is expensive, risky, and time-consuming. As such, companies are most likely to invest in products for which a strong return on investment is likely, such as drugs that treat long-term, chronic illnesses, lifestyle issues, and products that benefit people in developed countries who can afford to pay for them. Most antiinfectives, particularly antibiotics, which are used for short durations (7-14 days), face restricted use to avoid the development of resistance, resistance limits effectiveness and profitability, etc.; vaccines; and medicines desperately needed in the developing world are being left out.

Spurring Infectious Diseases Product Research and Development

Policymakers and the public should have no illusions that future pharmaceutical charity will be sufficient to address the existing and emerging infectious pathogens that threaten U.S. and global health. Instead, IDSA believes the burden is on the federal government to entice industry to antiinfective R&D as a means to protect U.S. public health and strengthen national security.

Robust R&D programs are needed to respond successfully to existing infectious diseases as well as new threats on the horizon. Market forces alone will not solve the current crisis in infectious diseases drug, vaccine and diagnostic R&D—that's why we need innovative public policy changes such as those that have been contemplated in the "Infectious Diseases Research and Development Act", a bipartisan bill introduced by Rep. Barbara Cubin last year. IDSA has strongly endorsed this bill and is particularly grateful to Rep. Cubin's commitment in this area. We encourage the Subcommittee to consider the bill as it moves forward to reauthorize Project Bioshield.

The "Infectious Diseases Research and Development Act" will provide incentives for pharmaceutical companies and biotechnology companies to invest in research and development with respect to antibiotic drugs, antivirals, diagnostic tests, and vaccines that may be used to identify, treat, or prevent *a "qualified infectious disease product."*

The bill defines a "*qualified infectious disease product*" as "any antibiotic drug, antiviral, diagnostic test, or vaccine that is developed for the purpose of treating, detecting, preventing, or identifying…an infectious pathogen identified by the [new] Commission [on Infectious Diseases Product Development, discussed below.]"

Prior to the establishment of the Commission and its initial report of infectious pathogens, the incentives outlined in the bill will be available in the interim to infectious diseases products addressing the following issues:

- methicillin-resistant staphylococcus areus—can infect the heart, bones, lungs, and bloodstream.
- life-threatening gram negative bacteria including, among others:
    - *Acinetobacter*, a type of bacteria that has caused stubborn wound infections in at 100 U.S. solders and civilians stationed in Iraq, and is an increasing cause of pneumonia in U.S. hospitals.
    - *Escherichia coli* and *Klebsiella* species, which are major causes of urinary tract, gastrointestinal tract, and wound infections.
- influenza–of particular note, the bill would entice the manufacture of products to treat influenza within the United States borders—an urgent need.
- Additional infectious pathogens as may be identified by the Secretary of Health and Human Services (HHS), in concurrence with infectious diseases clinicians.

As noted above, the bill establishes the Commission on Infectious Diseases Product Development. The Commission is required to identify the most dangerous infectious disease pathogens and their associated diseases that are or are likely to become a danger to public health. The Commission would provide an annual report to Congress, the President, and the Secretary of Health and Human Services (HHS) on its findings, conclusions, and recommendations, including an updated list of emerging infectious pathogens.

Not later than 90 days after the date of enactment of the bill, the Commission also would be required to report recommendations on the actions the Secretary of HHS should take to ensure that a sufficient quantity of vaccines and anti-virals are available to treat the American population in the event of a pandemic influenza outbreak.

The Commission would be comprised of 19 voting members appointed by the President; 12 members to be appointed from among the leading representatives of the infectious disease medical, research, pharmaceutical, and biological communities, 7 members from the general public; additional nonvoting members would be appointed from the leading federal health agencies.

The Cubin bill also includes several incentives to spur R&D for qualified infectious diseases products that IDSA supports. Pathogens/diseases identified by the Commission as priorities for action would be eligible for these incentives. IDSA supports that following incentives:

- Full restoration of patent terms to account for the time lost during FDA review of a new drug application.
- Fast-track FDA review of designated qualified infectious diseases products.
- Intensified efforts to assist small businesses in conducting end-stage clinical trials through NIH small business awards.
- Tax Credits for R&D: Allows manufacturers of qualified infectious diseases products to take a tax credit equal to 35% of the qualified infectious diseases research expenses for the taxable year.
- Manufacturing Facilities Investment Tax Credit: Provides a tax credit of 20% for a facility that is used for manufacturing, distributing, or for research and development of a qualified infectious diseases product.
- Clinical Trial Guidelines for Antibiotic Drugs: Requires the FDA to issue guidelines, within one year, for the conduct of clinical trials with respect to antibiotic drugs, including antimicrobials to treat resistant pathogens, bacterial meningitis, acute bacterial sinusitis, acute bacterial otitis media, and acute exacerbation of chronic bronchitis.

To strengthen the bill further, IDSA would encourage the following incentives be considered:

- FDA Priority Review Voucher—Under this concept, a voucher would be provided to a company that obtains an approval for a "qualified product" that treats a disease identified by the Commission. The company could then apply the voucher to a separate product (i.e., a potential blockbuster) of its choosing or, alternatively, the company could auction the voucher to another company. The voucher concept was raised in the March/April 2006 edition of Health Affairs. The authors say that this concept may reduce FDA's review time of a product by a year, which could be worth "more than $300 million for a potential blockbuster". Even if the FDA review time was reduced only by 6 months, IDSA believes this concept would have merit. A significant advantage of this approach is that it would not extend the length of the patent. As such, it should not be a threat to the generics industry. Instead, it would permit a company to market a product months in advance of when it otherwise would. This also would be an advantage to patients as they would be able to enjoy the product's benefits sooner. The Health Affairs articles authors report the cost of changing FDA's review from standard to priority review may be $1 million, which could be recovered through a user fee by the voucher user. Of note, under the authors' approach, the company would have to forgo patent rights—this is an idea that IDSA does not support.

- Extension of Patent Term for Qualified Infectious Diseases Products—Although fraught with politics, the extension of the patent term of critical needed qualified infectious diseases products for 2 years or even 6 months is one sure way to pique industry's interest. There are so few solutions available to address the lackluster pharmaceutical pipeline for antibiotics and other antiinfectives. It may be time for Congress to consider this idea.
- Tax Credits for R&D—IDSA would suggest increasing the amount of the tax credit for R&D in the Cubin bill to 50% to mirror the amount provided to orphan drugs under the Orphan Drug Act. IDSA also would suggest applying this tax credit to preclinical research as well as product clinical research and development.
- Protocol Assistance—In addition to the development of clinical guidelines by FDA, we also would support the agency's provision of additional protocol assistance similar to what is provided with regard to orphan drugs.
- Waiver of User Fees—We would support the waiver of all user fees related to FDA review of qualified infectious diseases products.
- Antitrust exemptions—additional flexibility for certain company communications is needed.
- Guaranteed Market—While it can be loosely argued that Project Bioshield may be applied already to naturally occurring resistant organisms, it is not likely that the Administration will view such infections as priorities unless Congress strengthens its emphasis in this area.
- Funding for CDC's Antimicrobial Resistance Program—Although it may be outside the scope of the Subcommittee's reauthorization effort, we appeal to you to help strengthen CDC's resistance program so that the agency may better lead the nation to respond to the silent epidemic that antimicrobial resistance has created. A multi-pronged approach is essential to limit the impact of antibiotic resistance on patients and public health. For this reason IDSA supports *a $25 million increase in this program to a total commitment of $50 million in FY 2007.* This will enable CDC to expand its surveillance of clinical and prescribing data that are associated with drug-resistant infections, to gather morbidity and mortality data due to resistance, to educate physicians and parents about the need to protect the long-term effectiveness of antibiotics, and to strengthen infection control activities across the United States. Broadening the number of CDC's extramural grants in applied research at academic-based centers also would harness the brainpower of our nation's researchers.

Conclusion

The reauthorization of Project Bioshield provides a critical opportunity to spur the development of new tools to protect Americans and the global community against the scourge of infectious diseases, particularly antibiotic resistant organisms, and bioterrorism. We urge congressional leaders to show bold leadership as it renews this legislation.

Specific to antibiotics, the past two decades of antibiotic development clearly have demonstrated that we no longer can rely on existing market forces to keep companies engaged in this area of drug discovery and development. Should additional companies' antibiotic R&D infrastructures be dismantled, it will take years to establish new programs—or this expertise could simply be lost forever. New antibiotics are desperately needed to treat serious as well as common infections. The bacteria that cause these infections are becoming increasingly resistant to the antibiotics that for years have been considered standard of care, and the list of resistant pathogens keeps growing. It is not possible to predict when an epidemic of drug-resistant bacteria will occur—but we do know it will happen.

Drugs, vaccines and diagnostics also are needed across the spectrum of infectious diseases medicine, including to address the growing threat of pandemic influenza. Conquering AIDS, TB, malaria, the neglected diseases found primarily in developing countries, and the next emerging infection will require renewed vision, creative policymaking and righteous action.

We appreciate the opportunity to testify. We look forward to working with you in the coming months to develop federal legislation to spur the tools infectious diseases physicians need to treat our seriously ill patients. Thank you.

MR. DEAL. Thank you. Very interesting testimony. Let me start with a few of the issues that each of you sort of touched on. Mr. Wright, you said that the first principle that you would suggest to us is clarity in establishing a central authority, and in my earlier questions to the first panel, I sort of overviewed the relationship and the roles DOD, Homeland Security, and HHS each play in the current structure. Are you suggesting by this recommendation that the current bifurcation of those functions is not appropriate and should be consolidated, is that what you are saying?

DR. WRIGHT. Yes, sir, the Alliance believes that the way it is currently being done, there are just too many players involved with too many different agendas, and there is not a clear person or place that Congress can go to and say, why don't we have this? It goes from one to the other. The DOD actually has a process that is much clearer and has worked for years in the procurement of products which there are no other markets for.

MR. DEAL. If you were to recommend where you think that consolidation should occur, do you have any recommendations?

DR. WRIGHT. Boy, that is a loaded question. No, I really don't. I actually think it probably belongs in the NIH as a separate committee.

MR. DEAL. Have any of the panel members had any opportunity to compare the different methods that are used, the DOD process versus the HHS process, with respect to countermeasure development? And if you have had that opportunity to observe the two approaches, do you have any comments you would like to make about those?

MR. COHEN. Mr. Chairman, if you are speaking of through DOD, I could speak to the way DARPA does it, which is very different from the way HHS does it. In a previous company, we were able to secure a multi-year commitment from DARPA for a countermeasure; it was an antibiotic. It was a fast process that involved the submission a rather modestly sized white paper that they used to compare the applications to, and was followed by a very large grant application. But the key difference was that the money was committed for three years, subject to ability to meet certain milestones, and we took that award and turned essentially a $6 million grant into about $50 million of private equity capital. That was very helpful to us raising money to build a program.

Within HHS and NIH in particular, you have to do very complicated grant applications that can be for as little as $200,000, and then a year later you get to apply for more money and each process takes a year. It has uncertainty related to the peer review process and also the appropriations process, and so you can't take those awards to investors and say I am going to take part of the risk off your shoulders and put it on the Government's. So that ability of the Defense Department, through DARPA at least, to give you a commitment subject to your meeting certain milestones makes a huge difference in our ability to raise what is substantial outside capital.

MR. DEAL. Which was the model that you suggested in your testimony?

MR. COHEN. Yes.

MR. DEAL. Mr. Young.

MR. YOUNG. This doesn't presume to make a structural or organizational recommendation and, to the little bit of familiarity I have with how DOD historically has approached vaccine development, I am not sure that that is the model I would recommend. But I think what it does suggest, from an industry's perspective, you would approach this with three paramount criteria in mind. You would want people involved who had an intimate understanding and experience level in the objective in question, which is actually practical development of products. There are wonderful people, expert scientists, dedicated and experienced civil servants and public health officials that inhabit many of these agencies, but there aren't many people who have actually developed products successfully in an industry setting, and that is a time consuming, very sophisticated process that requires a lot of judgment and the ability to handle a constantly evolving landscape towards a reasonably certain and clear ultimate product target.

On that point, I think what is clearly missing now is something to address the compartmentalization. You can get early stage funding, you can get late stage procurement support, but there is no coherent integrated picture of the whole development process that is evident to an industry participant in the effort. Thank you.

MR. DEAL. Thank you. Mr. Wright, my time is up, so maybe someone else will pursue this further. Ms. Eshoo, you are recognized for questions.

MS. ESHOO. Thank you, Mr. Chairman, and I want to thank all the panelists. I think that you have done an excellent job and you have also set some of the seeds popping in my mind. I think, first of all, and this is an observation, Mr. Chairman and my colleagues that are here today for this hearing, I think what is lacking in all of this is a real sense of urgency, and, Dr. O'Toole, you spoke so eloquently to that. There is a rhetoric war, and we know it and we hear it, and there is urgency to it. There isn't in this program. If we were to parse out in the Department of Defense whether there should be tanks or munitions or whatever, there would be a great deal of dissention in the Congress and in the country over that, and yet we are doing that with a program that deserves the same kind of defense, so to speak. We have now lived through and witnessed the disorganization within a Government agency, Homeland Security, in response to Katrina, and I can't help but think that we are not prepared. We are not prepared if, God forbid, any of these catastrophes were to be visited upon the United States. And so I think more than anything else, the way for the committee to approach this is with a great sense of urgency. If, in fact, we do that, then it is not going to be--and I am paraphrasing Dr. O'Toole--a stockpile of medicines. It is going to be larger than that.

The second point I want to make here and what I have learned from the panelists is, is that whatever dollars are in the pot, the Federal pot, they are really not being used as the right kind of magnet for the private sector to develop what needs to be developed. It is not working. I mean, there is the valley of death, all the other things that have been described. So the opportunity costs for the private sector are just too great in order for them to be attracted to do anything relative to this effort. So I think in some ways we are kidding ourselves. I think the program is aptly named, but it seems to kind of fall apart after that, and I am not saying that the people involved in it are not earnest. They are solid public servants, they want to do the right job. I think this committee, Mr. Chairman, needs to begin to redirect this. The whole notion that the Government is the only customer, we need to understand that, and that the companies are not going to engage in, as Bruce Cohen said, the companies are simply not going to be able to engage in it. Especially small companies, biotech companies, are not going to be able to engage in this, because they don't have the capital to do it. So if we don't capitalize on the issue that is before us with a great sense of urgency, then I think we are going to have a lot more hearings with reports that don't have the sense of urgency that they need to have.

Now, anyone who wants to chime in, I mean I am putting the ball in your court, but I think your testimony has been outstanding, and I think that you have, for me at least, struck a match here and cast some light on it. I think this needs to be revisited in a very serious way. How much more funding do you think is appropriate in this program? Anyone from the panel, Dr. O'Toole?

DR. O'TOOLE. I think we are off by about a magnitude of order, so ten times as much. But you know, part of the problem, I think you are right, one does not perceive this sense of urgency when you are looking at the HHS program from the outside. Part of the problem is that the urgency, the need to get something in the stockpile fast, is at war with the complexity--

MS. ESHOO. Yes.

DR. O'TOOLE. --of creating new drugs and figuring out what drugs we ought to be buying for the stockpile and what we ought to be investing in, in the future. These are new problems for the Government and they are new problems for the world. There isn't a prototype out there for how to do this. So HHS is in the position of inventing new processes for high stakes decisions, you know--

MS. ESHOO. Is that what the plan was that was alluded to or mentioned earlier from the first panel?

DR. O'TOOLE. That was the first I have heard of the strategic plan. It is a good idea to have a strategic plan.

MS. ESHOO. But it is the first you have heard of it?

DR. O'TOOLE. Yes.

MS. ESHOO. So you all are the modern day defense contractors. I think that is the way we have to think of this. I think that is the way we need to be thinking of this. Yes.

DR. BLASER. I would like to mention, from the standpoint of the Infectious Diseases Society, we also believe it should not be business as usual. We have to move things up a magnitude.

MS. ESHOO. Yes.

DR. BLASER. I am reminded of two analogies. One is the Manhattan Project where $2 billion in 1940 dollars were given for a major problem in national security. We were fighting a war then. In today's dollars, that is probably $20 billion. I think that is the scale we should think about. The other analogy is Katrina. We know that hurricanes occur, we don't know when, but we have to build up the infrastructure to protect us. In most years, the levees don't do us any good, but when we need them, we need them, and antibiotic resistance is the level of the water rising and influenza is the big storm. So when we put those together, we need to have that infrastructure of research and development for bioterrorism, for flu, for antibiotic resistance. They are all related.

MS. ESHOO. Bruce, did you want to say something?

MR. YOUNG. I would just add that there is another underlying difficulty here for the Government, is how does the Government bet on innovation?

MS. ESHOO. Yes.

MR. YOUNG. It is intrinsically risky. The way the private sector does this, it expects, it knows that within a portfolio of effort, it is going to have failure. I think it is very difficult in this climate to spend this kind of money and not say, what are we getting for the money, when you can predict that a significant percentage of what you are going to get is a dry well. But if you don't do that, if you don't have a culture and an approach and a willingness to embrace the risk, you will get no change, no improvement, no innovation.

MR. COHEN. I would like to speak to Congresswoman Eshoo's point about the defense analogy. Right now, we are stuck in a place where you can either get a very tiny and insignificant amount of money, or you have to bet on a $700 million contract, and that isn't the way the defense industry basically built Silicon Valley. At least those of us from California know that you make relatively modest sized grants and contracts, you take lots of bets, and we are not talking about tens of millions of dollars, but that enables people to go do interesting innovation. But it also, as we have learned, draws private capital in, and the system right now is not drawing private capital because it is too unpredictable and the amounts of money are in the extreme, they are not in the middle. And that can be changed. It is not that hard to do that. Some of us have products that have crossover applications and some don't, but regardless of the degree to which there is a so-called civilian application for what you are doing, the ability to get the private capital into the game is really essential and that can be fixed.

MR. DEAL. Thank you. Very interesting question and comments.

MS. ESHOO. Thank you, Mr. Chairman.

MR. DEAL. Mr. Shimkus?

MR. SHIMKUS. Thank you, Mr. Chairman. And if we have accomplished one thing, we have struck Anna Eshoo's match and as I know from past activities, when you do that, you really do get a response. I will just go back to our E-911 aspect. She was complaining about the fact that you couldn't find people years before it became a d' jour item, and now we are almost getting to a point where with your cell phone, people now know where you are at. And I don't want to harangue my colleagues, but you know, look at this committee hearing room. You know, you have interested Members, but we ought to have more here if it is that serious of an issue and we don't and so that is part of the dilemma. I always talk about raising capital. Really, most businesses borrow, go to the private equity markets, go to Wall Street, assume a risk, hoping to get a rate of return. Well, you all are doing it for hopefully no consumers. I mean, in a perfect world, we have the ability to respond, but we never have to use it, and so then that is the ultimate risk. All this money poured out and no return, so that is far as I read it, that is this valley of death and how do you bridge that. And you know, Mr. Cohen, I really appreciated your comments, because there has got to be a way if we addressed a couple things.

By centralizing this whole operation, maybe we can target individual grants, which then would incur private capital and you leverage that, and we do that on water projects, in fact, you almost want that, because you want people empowered to it. You just don't want the Federal government doing it. You want to incentivize other folks. And I think we have a problem with this monetary debate. We need a magnitude of 10. Well, a magnitude of ten of what, the $5 billion that we have authorized but have only spent one, or $50 billion, $50 billion or, as I have come to know, we have got $5 billion now, but we have got $2 billion in the NIH budget, we have got DOD dollars, so I think there is a lot of money out there. But, because we are not centralized, we are not maybe effectively using it or at least we don't know where it is at.

But you have brought up a lot of good debate for us to get our hands on this, because the public is just not going to accept our response that we had a hearing and the country is not prepared to respond. Dr. Cohen, I don't want to get off on an issue, but I am also interested in knowing where do your adult stem cells come from?

MR. COHEN. In the case of the part that we are talking about for nuclear countermeasures, they come from donors.

MR. SHIMKUS. I mean, is it blood, is it teeth, is it adult fat, tissues, where?

MR. COHEN. It is called mobilized peripheral blood and we pay people to essentially donate blood and we extract stem cells from that.

MR. SHIMKUS. Now, in just using that as an example, one of the concerns is, as I mentioned before, how do you have an antidote or a drug for immediate application? What is infectious time? And then, is there a debate on how you can rapidly create it? Do we have to have a stockpile of all this stuff or, through research and development, can we have dispersed sites that can rapidly deploy and make antidotes in a timely manner? I mean, I don't know. I am not a doctor. So, in your field, which is radiology and the aspects, do you have to have stuff on hand?

MR. COHEN. Well, first of all, I am not a doctor, either, but in the treatment of radiological injury, because we treat those patients when they undergo chemotherapy or radiation therapy, we know a lot about the time between exposure and when you have to treat.

MR. SHIMKUS. And that is why you have a private application which people are willing to invest capital in?

MR. COHEN. That is right. And so what it appears from the animal models that we have done, and I think clinical experience is you can imagine the national stockpile some place in a cave where it is safe, where you could store enough doses that you get to the affected area within, say, four to seven days. And if you use a cell-based medicine, which is a regenerative therapy, then you have the ability to wait that much more time before you treat the patients, so you don't have to have it deployed in their house, and that is only for radiological injury. What would happen in practice is that they would be stored frozen, and it appears, based on perhaps 30 years of experience, that this, a cellular product, is safe for at least a decade in a frozen state. Then you would have it transported to the site of the incident, and it would be administered by the kinds of people who work as emergency medical technicians in ambulances who can do simple infusions. In animal models, this rescues a substantial number of animals, not everybody, because sometimes you get too much radiation and nothing works and there is some population, and the Government has this all sort of worked out, what the radiological dose would be. Some people would survive with basic antibiotic therapy. Some people wouldn't survive. We are focused on the middle of people who are rescuable but otherwise wouldn't, and I think the only real live experience of that is Chernobyl, and most of the people at Chernobyl died of what is called hematopoietic failure, too many of their stem cells died to populate their immune system, and we know pretty certainly you can replace that with a cell-based medicine and you should have enough time to get there.

MR. SHIMKUS. And I appreciate that. It just highlights one other question I was going to ask and I am just going to throw it out there. I still think that in the previous panel, Mr. Chairman, they talked about the local health providers being able to, then ramp up the thing in the local health providers. Well, if you have a nuclear explosion in a major metropolitan area, that is similar to a Katrina, where you just overwhelm the local providers and that is where the national debate, and I know we have got this issue about the military intervening. But I am an Army infantry airborne guy, so you parachute the 82nd in, they set up their field hospitals, they receive the drugs and then they try to do that in an expedited manner, which is more efficient than if you try to cobble together the first-line responders who, in a large geographical area, could be all gone and that still has got to be part of this debate. And I do agree with, again, my colleague, Anna Eshoo, we should take the lead and even though it is not hip and not cool, but we ought to pursue this, Mr. Chairman, and I thank you for the hearing and I yield back.

MR. DEAL. I thank the gentleman. Dr. Burgess.

MR. BURGESS. Thank you, Mr. Chairman. And you know, the timeline that is before us with, say, avian flu is something none of us can know, but there is reasonable evidence that, because of the migratory flyways, this hemisphere could see its first outbreak in northern Canada midsummer, August, in the southern tier of Canadian provinces, and three weeks before Election Day in East Texas and Georgia. So it is not just a theoretic application that we are talking about here, and we do need to be prepared. And it is difficult to get Congress mobilized, but I appreciate your efforts in this hearing to do that.

Dr. Wright, I will just say I sympathize with you when you told the Chairman that the whole process was too diffuse, and there was no jurisdiction. You can imagine my surprise of getting to here that there was no committee on health that I could join. I looked around for it for a long time, but I finally found a home here on Energy and Commerce and I was grateful for it. But even amongst our subcommittee, we have division of labor with some other committees and it does make inherently difficult to do at the congressional level. And at the same time, the world is a menacing place and we do need to be able to move with a great deal more facility, and I do appreciate the comments of all of you today. Ms. Eshoo spoke about the urgency. Unfortunately, the urgency may be provided for us, and I hope that is not the case, but certainly there are scenarios that are being modeled out there right with computer simulation that dictate that there may be more urgency to the avian flu than any one of us would like to admit.

Dr. Blaser, I was intrigued by one of the comments you made about the antibiotic-resistant bacteria and how, perhaps, one of the tools at your disposal might be to lengthen the time in patent for development of some antibiotics and I wondered if you had some additional thoughts for us about that.

DR. BLASER. The urgent need is to develop new antibiotics for resistant organisms. That is where our great focus is and our recommendation, which is completely consistent with Representative Cubin's bill, is to develop a national commission that will recommend to HHS situations in which we need to develop qualified products. And for those qualified products, for those targeted areas, then we would offer a package of incentives to bring our industrial, our biotech, and our small and big companies back into the marketplace so that it is economically viable. We are interested in a variety of approaches, including tax credits, including expedited review, including patent extension for those qualified products.

MR. BURGESS. But those things wouldn't necessarily just be under the purview of Project BioShield, right? Those are for any drug out there on the development horizon.

DR. BLASER. Well again, our interest is in what we would call these qualified products. They could be for pandemic influenza as part of the pandemic flu preparedness, it could be for antibiotic resistance, it could be for bioterrorism. Right now, under BioShield, there is an apparatus in terms of the Government being a single supplier, but listening to the testimony today, I am impressed by the need to have middle level kinds of support, not tiny ones and not the mammoth ones, but develop a very broad pipeline. Now that is our strength in America and we can't predict exactly where the great innovation is coming from. We need to seed it broadly.

MR. BURGESS. Well, Mr. Cohen, in your discussions of your product to protect people from radiation, from the hematopoietic syndrome, it sounds to me like you are talking about the Phase III trials that your company is finding difficult to getting funding. Is that correct?

MR. COHEN. No, in our case, we can't get the Phase I trials funded, so--

MR. BURGESS. You are getting some help from NIH?

MR. COHEN. We have grants from NIH for preclinical research. And while, technically, NIH can fund clinical trials, it doesn't, and BioShield doesn't, and those trials cost several million dollars which, for a company of my size, is a substantial amount of money.

MR. BURGESS. I thought it cost several hundred million dollars, in actuality. Is that not correct?

MR. COHEN. Not necessarily. So the Phase I trials are several million dollars and the Phase II trials can be perhaps ten times that.

MR. BURGESS. Right.

MR. COHEN. BioShield can, under the current law, you can get approved without a definitive Phase III trial, particularly if the application is to something you can't test for.

MR. BURGESS. I see, okay.

MR. COHEN. So we may not be needing to go to this sort of gigantic trial that people contemplate in our industry, typically, so I don't think we are talking about that. And if we were going to do a trial that big, it would probably be because we had a private market, and then that would be something private investors would pay for.

MR. BURGESS. So they could absorb some of it. Yes, Dr. Wright?

DR. WRIGHT. However, in a vaccine, even in BioShield, you are going to be looking at 2,000, 3,000, 5,000 patients in a Phase I safety trial. We are developing a product for anthrax. We are right now, we have finished our first Phase I trial. We are in the process of having to go to scale-up. There is no RFP. There is no commitment to buy. We don't know how much the Government will buy. Our venture capital partners are backing out from funding us because there is no market, there is no active RFP, and the company needs to spend $12 million to do a tech transfer in a scale-up to be ready to manufacture it so we can do our final proof of principal trials. We are not alone in that. This is a scenario of every company in this industry. It runs from a scale of $20 million to probably $300 million that is needed to fund this middle area. But also what is needed is to know on the end that there is a market for your product. There has got to be an RFP out there saying, hey, if you do this, we will buy your product, otherwise, venture, the street, and private capital will not come in. That is missing from the current BioShield legislation.

MR. BURGESS. Thank you, Mr. Chairman. I will yield back.

MR. DEAL. Mrs. Cubin.

MRS. CUBIN. Thank you, Mr. Chairman. I was taken by your testimony, Dr. O'Toole, when you said what I believe to have been that stockpiling isn't the only answer, and I certainly believe it isn't the only answer. So I wonder, do you think that methodology--and I am speaking in reference to R and D done on antibiotic, new antibiotics like we have talked about a little bit and that Dr. Blaser talked about that my bill would help facilitate development of. Do you think that methodology or a new research-type roadmap or something produced through the R and D on mutated microorganisms could be used to find countermeasure development treatments for bioengineered weapons? In other words, you know, it seems to me that what we learned from treating these mutated microorganisms, if we found the gene in MRSA, for example, that caused it to mutate, could that information be translated and used to help develop potential treatments for bioweapons?

DR. O'TOOLE. Well, increasing the store of biological knowledge and knowing better how the parts and circuits of living organisms work is going to help us across the board. In dealing with bioengineered organisms, we are going to have a number of strategies that we are going to have to choose between. It may be that some drugs that we never thought of using against, for example, antibiotic-resistant anthrax or a new kind of engineered virus, would work against this biological weapon, but we would have to be able to screen those drugs against the weapon very carefully. We could set up a kind of consortium of rapid throughput screening and have library banks of current drugs that we could turn to in an emergency, if we wanted to do that. That would require cooperation amongst the many drug companies who own those databanks. We might be able to develop therapies that would boost immune response at least for an interim period of time, not necessarily like Mr. Cohen's product does, but along the same lines. You could get a kind of generic boost to the immune system to help tide people over and get them through acute stages. Or you might, in the future, if we were very successful and very ambitious, be able to come up with new drugs in very short periods of time, tailor made to fit the bioengineered drug. My point is the Nation is going to have to undertake a strategy of radical acceleration of drug development to deal with this threat. If you do that, you are going to decrease the cost of drug development generally, which is going to have enormous benefits for the cost of healthcare, et cetera. I think the problem will be forced upon us either by a pandemic flu, maybe of a strain that we do not have a vaccine for, or by a bioattack. I think it will come and we are going to have to take it on. It would be better if we did it before such a calamity befell us.

MRS. CUBIN. Well, and it seems to me that there could be not a direct appropriation from the Government, but an influx of private investment, if the advantages that are in my bill that Dr. Blaser spoke about were made available to pharmaceutical companies. Dr. Blaser, are naturally occurring drug-resistant diseases being overlooked by current biothreat preparedness today?

DR. BLASER. It is a little hard for me to answer that question, so I may answer it a little differently and say that we could think that there are three threats in front of us, bioterrorism, pandemic and regular influenza, and antibiotic resistance. We can just take these as three major threats, and for each of these, we have to develop vaccinology, antivirals, antibiotics, and new diagnostics, and there is tremendous crossover between these fields. As Dr. O'Toole said, what we do in bioterrorism vaccinology will help us in influenza and vice versa, and so, in many ways, we see these natural or manmade threats as a continuum. And like Dr. O'Toole, we think, even though the country is scaling up, it is probably not scaling up enough, and we wouldn't necessarily propose to take away from bioterrorism to put into the other. We think this pie has to be enlarged and if we don't do it, it is going to cost us much more later.

MRS. CUBIN. I certainly agree with that, and I certainly don't think my bill by any means is the only solution. I think it is a piece to an enormous puzzle. I would like the rest of you to respond, if you would, on how you think a bill like what you have heard described without holding you to it, since you haven't read the details. But theoretically, do you think that that could fold into, help with BioShield, and do you think that this problem that we are addressing in that bill would actually fold into--even though I understand that is not what BioShield does, but should it, should we be considering these resistant drugs and the mutation of resistant microorganisms and other mutated microorganisms?

DR. WRIGHT. I think from the Alliance perspective, we have discussed this a lot; where does infectious disease and biodefense overlap. And there is a tremendous overlap, and it is very hard to rule out one having an effect on the other. We believe that the technology involved in infectious disease can do nothing but help with the biodefense products that are needed to be developed, especially in the area of engineered biodefense or bioterrorism products. And so that is when someone takes anthrax and makes it antibiotic resistant. That is when this type of bill and the technology could really help out events.

MRS. CUBIN. Mr. Young.

MR. YOUNG. Thank you. I have an industry infectious disease background, it is a little stale, but I think what I would say on this is that it sounds to me like a bill that supports the effort to identify new technology targets is all to the good so you have a pipeline of new scientific insights coming to bear that can be used to develop practical applications. My concern, however, is that I think the experience of BioShield so far to date is that the agencies involved have insufficient focus on the practical requirements of product development where there are some product opportunities a little further down the pipeline in the development pathway. NIH has experience in early stage research. They have migrated laterally into product development, but that expertise is still substantially undeveloped and we have talked a lot about the coordination to try and fill the gaps, the funding to support the gaps, to move the product opportunities along. So I would agree with the perspective that says this is a big puzzle, it is woefully underfunded, and that what you are describing should be a piece of the puzzle.

MRS. CUBIN. Mr. Cohen, did I see you raise your hand? Okay. Dr. O'Toole.

DR. O'TOOLE. I would just say that a drug-resistant bacteria makes a great weapon.

MRS. CUBIN. Thank you. Thank you, Mr. Chairman.

MR. DEAL. Thank you. And thanks to the very distinguished panel. Your testimony, I think, has added greatly to our consideration of the reauthorization of this legislation. We thank you, and with that, this hearing is adjourned.

[Whereupon, at 3:25 p.m., the subcommittee was adjourned.]

RESPONSE FOR THE RECORD BY THE HON. ALEX M. AZAR, DEPUTY SECRETARY, U.S. DEPARTMENT OF HEALTH AND HUMAN SERVICES

The Honorable Tom Allen
Questions for The Honorable Alex M. Azar. Deputy Secretary
U.S. Department of Health and Human Services
April 6, 2006
Subcommittee on Health
Hearing entitled: "Project Bioshield Reauthorization Issues"

1. **Take a hypothetical case where the Secretary determines that the most effective countermeasure to an emerging bio-threat is being developed overseas by a foreign-owned manufacturer. What barriers, if any, are there to the procurement of such a countermeasure produced overseas?**

   As provided by the Project BioShield Act of 2004, security countermeasures are drugs, biological products, or devices (as defined under the FD&C Act) which are among other things, (1) approved or cleared, or (2) have sufficient and satisfactory clinical experience or research data to support a reasonable conclusion that the countermeasures will qualify for approval or licensing within 8 years, or (3) are authorized for emergency use under section 564 of the FD&C Act. While the Federal Government would prefer to obtain medical countermeasures from domestic sources due to the inherent risks involved in product development, imported products manufactured in foreign FDA-inspected facilities that meet the criteria established by Project BioShield are eligible for BioShield procurement.

   Generally speaking, medical countermeasures produced by foreign manufacturers may be legally imported into the U.S. if they are FDA-approved, licensed, or cleared, if they are under an investigational new drug application (IND) or an investigational device exemption (IDE), or are authorized for emergency use, and if they are otherwise in compliance with the FD&C Act. These legal standards also apply to domestically produced countermeasures.

2. **The Project BioShield Act allows for the purchase of unapproved and unlicensed countermeasures if the Secretary determines there is a reasonable conclusion that the product would be approved and licensed. The Act also allows the Secretary to authorize use of medical products that have not been approved by the FDA or HHS if emergency circumstances merit.**

   a.) Does the authority under this Act, or any other Act, also allow for the import of medical products to meet an emergency need if there is no domestic source?

   As provided by the Project BioShield Act of 2004, security countermeasures are drugs, biological products, or devices (as defined under the FD&C Act) which are among other things, (1) approved or cleared, or (2) have sufficient and satisfactory clinical experience or research data to support a reasonable conclusion that the countermeasures will qualify for approval or licensing within 8 years, or (3) are authorized for emergency use under section 564 of the FD&C Act. While the Federal Government would prefer to obtain medical countermeasures from domestic sources due to the inherent risks involved in product development, imported products manufactured in foreign FDA-inspected facilities that meet the criteria established by Project BioShield are eligible for BioShield procurement. Generally speaking, medical countermeasures produced by foreign manufacturers may be legally imported into the U.S. if they are FDA-approved, licensed, or cleared, if they are under an investigational new drug application (IND) or an investigational device exemption (IDE), or are authorized for emergency use, and if they are otherwise in compliance with the FD&C Act. These legal standards also apply to domestically produced countermeasures.

b.) If so, does this authority supersede the requirement under the Medicine Equity and Drug Safety Act [MEDS] that the Secretary must certify that a reimportation of a pharmaceutical product will "pose no additional risk to the public's health and safety? "

The purpose of the Medicine Equity and Drug Safety Act (MEDS Act) is to provide a means for prescription drugs manufactured in the United States and exported to certain foreign countries to be reimported from those countries for sale to American consumers by any pharmacist or wholesaler. BioShield countermeasures are developed and purchased through contracts with the Federal Government for the purpose of safeguarding the homeland and are not available for commercial sale. Therefore, the provisions established in the MEDS Act are not relevant within the context of Project BioShield procurements. The Project BioShield Act of 2004 is a unique statutory provision that addresses the need for countermeasures that address chemical, biological, nuclear, and radiological (CBERN) threats.

3. What remedies does the U.S. government have if confronted with the case where the Secretary finds that the U.S. patent holder to a particular countermeasure has insufficient manufacturing capacity to produce a sufficient quantity of the product to meet a bio-threat?

As part of the BioShield award process, prior to the contract award, qualified experts from industry, academia, and government perform technical evaluation of BioShield proposals to ensure that contractors have suitable manufacturing capacity to meet strict government requirements. Prior to award, the government requests information from contractors concerning their current manufacturing capabilities, the proposed production plan, and the estimated manufacturing capacity available to expedite the manufacture of the specified doses of product in the event of a national emergency. A contract would not be awarded if it appeared that the applicant has insufficient capacity to deliver the needed product.

4. Take the case where the Secretary determines that there is insufficient domestic manufacturing capacity for a countermeasure to meet a bio-threat, but that there is sufficient capacity overseas to produce generic versions of the same countermeasure. Does the Secretary have the ability or the authority to import such countermeasures in such circumstance?

As noted in the answer to question one above, the BioShield Act does have provisions to obtain countermeasures from either domestic or foreign sources. The issue of manufacturing capacity is addressed in question three above. Products acquired under Project BioShield are solely for national security purposes. This program is focused on the development of new countermeasures - products for which generic versions generally would not exist.

O